After studying biological medicine at the Heilpraktikersschule in Solingen in Germany (1977), **Jan Dries** specialized in nutritional therapy in association with the Avicenna Health Centre in Genk. Since then he has met and worked with thousands of people in search of a better diet. Over the past five years he has treated more than 600 cancer patients with his 'Dries cancer diet', a technique that has gained him international renown.

A lecturer at the Academy of Natural Medicine in Bloemendaal, Amsterdam, Holland, for eight years, Jan Dries has since 1988 been the chairman of the Executive Board of the European Academy of Complementary Medicine in Antwerp and Ghent, in Belgium. He is also chairman of the Vegetarian Society and the New Life Society, vice-chairman of the Association of Naturopaths, and holds distinguished offices in a number of other associations.

Previously published works include fifteen books and more than a hundred pamphlets on the subject of health, all of which have achieved some repute. In addition to his painstaking research in the field of nutrition, he has also made important contributions to such disciplines as bioenergy, herbal and natural medicine, relaxation therapy and reflexology.

Translated into seven languages, this book reveals Jan Dries yet again as the complete master of nutritional theory and practice. He has managed to present in an accessible yet scientific way the means by which food combining may find general acceptance and utility, while simultaneously resolving many of the doubts and misunderstandings of past critics, and fulfilling a need felt by many aware people.

Inge Dries grew up in a family where the attention was focused on healthy food and a natural way of life. From her mother, she inherited the love for preparing food and her father taught her everything about dietary rules. As a graphic designer, she pays a lot of attention to the presentation of her dishes, all of which are composed according to the correct food combinations. With these 200 tasty dishes, Inge Dries helps the reader apply the food combinations in a simple and pleasant way.

					acids					starch			sugar		fat			protein		
		mushrooms	milk	vegetables	vegetables (lactic acid)	yoghurt – butter milk	tomato	vinegar – mustard	fruits – berries	vegetables rich in starch	potato	cereals – bread – pasta	fruit rich in sugar	sugar – honey	avocado – olive	butter – whipped cream	oil – fat – egg yolk	nuts – seeds – pips	cheese – cottage cheese	meat – fish – poultry
protein	meat – fish – poultry	✓	–	✓	–	–	✓	–	–	×	–	–	–	–	–	–	–	–	–	■
	cheese – cottage cheese	✓	–	✓	–	×	✓	–	✓	×	–	–	–	–	–	–	–	–	■	–
	nuts – seeds – pips	•	–	✓	✓	×	✓	–	✓	×	–	–	–	–	–	–	–	■	–	–
fat	oil – fat – egg yolk	✓	×	✓	✓	✓	✓	✓	✓	✓	✓	✓	×	–	–	–	■	–	–	–
	butter – whipped cream	✓	×	✓	✓	✓	✓	✓	✓	✓	✓	✓	×	–	–	■	–	–	–	–
	avocado – olive	✓	–	✓	✓	✓	✓	✓	✓	✓	✓	✓	–	–	■	–	–	–	–	–
sugar	sugar – honey	–	–	–	–	✓	•	•	✓	×	–	–	×	■	–	–	–	–	–	–
	fruit rich in sugar	–	–	–	–	✓	–	×	✓	×	–	–	■	×	–	×	×	–	–	–
starch	cereals – bread – pasta	✓	–	✓	–	–	–	–	–	✓	✓	■	–	–	✓	✓	✓	–	–	–
	potato	✓	–	✓	–	–	–	–	–	✓	■	✓	–	–	✓	✓	✓	–	–	–
	vegetables rich in starch	✓	–	✓	✓	✓	×	×	×	■	✓	✓	×	×	✓	✓	✓	×	×	×
acids	fruits – berries	–	×	×	×	✓	×	✓	■	×	–	–	✓	✓	✓	✓	✓	✓	✓	–
	vinegar – mustard	✓	×	✓	×	–	✓	■	✓	×	–	–	×	•	✓	✓	✓	–	–	–
	tomato	✓	×	✓	✓	✓	■	✓	×	×	–	–	–	•	✓	✓	✓	✓	✓	✓
	yoghurt – butter milk	•	✓	✓	✓	■	✓	–	✓	✓	–	–	✓	✓	✓	✓	✓	×	×	–
	vegetables (lactic acid)	✓	×	✓	■	✓	✓	×	×	✓	–	–	–	–	✓	✓	✓	✓	–	–
	vegetables	✓	×	■	✓	✓	✓	✓	×	✓	✓	✓	–	–	✓	✓	✓	✓	✓	✓
	milk	•	■	×	×	✓	×	×	×	–	–	–	–	–	–	×	×	–	–	–
	mushrooms	■	•	✓	✓	•	✓	✓	–	✓	✓	✓	–	–	✓	✓	✓	•	✓	✓

✓ good combinations × difficult combinations
– bad combinations • good, but not usual

The Food Combining Chart

The Complete Book of

Food Combining

*A New Approach to
Healthy Eating*

JAN DRIES
and
INGE DRIES

ELEMENT
Shaftesbury, Dorset • Boston, Massachusetts
Melbourne, Victoria

First published in Dutch under the titles *Voedselcombinaties* and 200 *Heerlijke gerechten*

First published in English by Element Books Limited under the titles *The New Book of Food Combining* and 200 *New Food Combining Recipes*

© Element Books Limited 1998
Text © Arinus 1992

This combined edition first published in the UK in 1998 by
Element Books Limited
Shaftesbury, Dorset SP7 8BP

Published in the USA in 1998 by
Element Books, Inc.
160 North Washington Street, Boston, MA 02114

Published in Australia in 1998 by
Element Books and distributed by
Penguin Australia Limited
487 Maroondah Highway, Ringwood, Victoria 3134

Reprinted June and December 1998

Cover design by Slatter-Anderson
Design by PPG Publishing Services
Typeset by PPG Publishing Services
Printed and bound in Great Britain by
J.W. Arrowsmith, Bristol

British Library Cataloguing in Publication
data available

Library of Congress Cataloging in Publication data

Dries. Jan.
    [voedselcumbinaries, English]
    The complete book of food combining new approach to healthy
eating / Jan Dries and Inge Dries. p.   cm.
    Originally published in 1995 as two separate works under the
titles, New book of food combining / Jan Dries, and, 200 new food
combining recipes / Inge Dries.
    Includes bibliographical references and index.
    1. food combining 2. Nutrition. I. Dries, Inge. 200 Heerlijke
gerechten, English. II. title.
    RA784 D7513 1998   613.2—dc21   97-45050 CIP

ISBN 1–86204–239–X

CONTENTS

FOREWORD

Food combining – the combining of specific foods for optimal digestive results – is a popular subject in today's world, promulgated in particular by the two well-known nutritionists Hay and Shelton. All the same, it would be wrong to try to make out that the theory behind such nutritional harmony is generally accepted. Only very recently in circles devoted to dietetics and health, for whom wholesome nutrition is the focus of all their efforts, has food combining and the study of the foods that are harmonious together received anything like its due interest.

People who still cannot accept the theory of food combining tend to assume that all foods contain basically the same nutrients, and that these nutrients are subject to the digestive processes simultaneously. Combining specific foods is thus a waste of time because 'all food goes down the same way'. Such people go on to point out that the principles on which Hay and Shelton based their work are somewhat behind the times in scientific terms, no longer corresponding to every concept of current physiological theory.

It was Jan Dries who, at least in Holland, during the 1970s greatly contributed to the revival of interest in food combining, waging what amounted almost to a personal crusade in publicizing and promoting the use of these important dietary combinations. His publications, his lectures, his course studies and his private correspondence have over the years led thousands of people into the way of health by means of food combining. And through research undertaken during those same years, he has since come up with further significant improvements.

With no disrespect at all to the highly creditable preliminary work carried out by Hay and Shelton, it would not be inaccurate to say that Jan Dries presents a completely new view of food combining. His extensive and thorough understanding of the physiology of digestion has at length furnished him with the answers to all the questions on food combining that scientists might wish to pose.

This brilliant book is a matchless guide to anyone who is searching for better and healthier nutrition.

Jef Houben
Biochemist

INTRODUCTION

In today's industrialized nations, the state of public health is nothing short of alarming. News broadcasts bring the dreadful truth home to us every day: the number of victims, the virulence of the diseases, the spread of the effects – all are getting worse as time goes on. Yet the causes are well known. They include the disruption of the environment, a stressful lifestyle, and a lack of purposive identity as a member of the organic species on the planet, and they also include the eating of food that has been produced and prepared by industrial methods. At the same time, health care has become so complex and (consequently) so disorganized that it verges on the unaffordable. The prospects are both terrifying and potentially tragic.

In northern Europe, North America and Australasia, humankind enjoys immense material benefits but must, ironically, even now fight for the preservation of its life more than ever. The three elements essential to that preservation and to future development – air, water, and food – correspond to the very elements most under threat in the environment.

For the last twenty years or so, considerable attention has been paid to promoting health foods, with particular emphasis on natural aspects. Organic cultivation has been encouraged not just by consumer demand but also by agricultural organizations and government food departments. The use of food additives has diminished rapidly. Many restaurants include a salad bar at which customers can select from a wide variety of raw vegetables. Vegetarianism is utterly accepted as a way of life.

But what is the point of all these positive developments if the food we choose is still not used to maximum advantage? Many of the people who turn to what should be a wholesome and nutritious diet find that they nonetheless continue to complain of digestive problems, a bloated feeling, and wind in the stomach and intestines, altogether comprising the sort of discomforts that they had hoped to eliminate once and for all. They thereupon lose all confidence in the idea of healthier nutrition, without realizing that they have just not made what they could of it.

Food combining, in which specific foods are combined for optimal digestive results, represents the solution for everyone: it works as well for those who stick to a conventional eating pattern as it does for those who have the willpower to opt for a less conventional but better one. Whatever we eat, we must always bear in mind exactly how the human digestive system functions. If we do not do that, not only is the digestion disrupted but the nutritional value that we get out of the food is minimal: we may eat plenty of food, but we do not make much use of it. This is a waste of food and energy. Moreover, it tends needlessly to clog up the intestines while also representing a burden to the liver and potentially causing the tissues to suffer some degree of acidosis. To go on eating huge quantities of food in this wasteful way is ironically to invite any of various deficiency conditions that are deleterious to overall health.

The more simple and natural is a person's eating pattern, the less is the need to practise food combining. This strongly indicates that those who follow a conventional eating pattern involving meat, fish, cheese, bread, and so forth, can benefit most from eating the recommended combinations of specific foods.

The main theme of this book is to demonstrate the value of food combining in relation to all eating patterns. The theory as formerly presented by the nutritionists Hay and Shelton may perhaps be rather past its sell-by date, but in this book the combinations of specific foods comply fully with the most advanced scientific views of modern physiology.

The principle behind food combining can be stated very simply. Every food contains up to five nutrients: proteins, fats, sugars, starch, and acids. Some nutrients are inert or passive in the presence of other nutrients – but some react with others, and cause disruption in the digestive process.

All foods contain these nutrients, and in proportions that are specific to each particular food. The nutrient that is proportionately the greatest in quantity (the dominant nutrient) 'programs' the entire digestive process. To eat different types of food at random may result in the presence of more than one dominant nutrient, and the consequent reaction between conflicting dominants may cause anything from a mild flush to serious digestive problems involving internal fermentation and gastroenteric poisoning.

Digestion relies primarily on the activity of enzymes that function within a fairly narrow range of acidity levels. Each type of food has an influence on the degree of acidity present, and can in turn influence the digestive process for better or for worse. Digestion is itself subject to circadian rhythms that are unfailingly strict on regular timing, and does not take well to random eating. Best, therefore, that a meal should comprise foods that are carefully suited to each other and that support each other as they are digested.

FOOD COMBINING CASE HISTORIES

Good food combining aids digestion and has a beneficial influence on total health and the healing process. The following are just five examples from the many thousands of people who have regained their health by using correct food combinations.

Jean, a forty-eight year old woman, suffered from shortness of breath. She took medicines and antibiotics over many years for bronchitis but they had no effect. Jan Dries noticed that her stomach and abdomen were bloated and were pushing up into her diaphragm causing respiratory problems. By adopting the right food combinations the swelling subsided and she was able to breathe normally.

John, a fifty-eight year old man, suffered from asthma. Once he began eating food in the right combinations, his asthma disappeared. When he did not pay attention to correct food combining, the asthma returned.

Frank, a thirty-two year old man, had epileptic fits. After he had adopted a good food combining regime, he no longer suffered from epilepsy. However, when he ate with his sister, who cooked traditional food in bad combinations, his attacks returned.

Sarah, a fifty-two year old woman, had problems with her intestines and bowels for many years. She was cured by eating small meals and using correct food combinations.

Karen, a twenty-four year old woman, suffered from psoriasis. She cut out all animal proteins from her diet and ate only good food combinations. As a result her psoriasis has healed.

This book is not meant to represent an apologia for the theory of food combining, but to emphasize the importance of a dietary regime that takes account of the theory's combinations of specific foods. It is an attempt to familiarize the reader with the necessary dietary rules. Above all, the book contains many tables, diagrams and lists, all of which are carefully annotated and explained. Using the correct combinations of specific foods in all meals should lead to virtually perfect digestion, maximum nutritional benefit, and total freedom from alimentary discomfort. As an added advantage, the body's whole metabolism should function at an optimum, with a consistently high degree of immunity from all sorts of ailments and diseases. Food combining is the first step to a healthy diet.

With this book I hope to convince as many people as possible that food combining is necessary for everyone and for every kind of eating pattern.

Enjoy your food!

Jan Dries

PART I
The Theory

CHAPTER 1

THE IMPORTANCE OF
FOOD COMBINING

Animals eat a simple diet that combines few nutrient types. Carnivores do not eat their carbohydrates in combination with proteins or acids. Ornithologists have noted that birds which eat insects at one particular time of the day may eat seeds at another time. The nut-nibbling squirrel eats no other food at all. Not one single wild animal eats such a great variety of foods as does civilized, industrialized humankind.

The enzymes of the human digestive system are subject to certain restrictions. If we eat in such a way as to cause these limitations to be exceeded, we suffer digestive problems. Good food combining is no more than a way of observing these enzymatic restrictions, to the benefit of our health. If we practise combining our food in the right manner, rather than just eating haphazardly, our digestion will be improved in efficiency and metabolic advantage.

We get nothing out of nutrients that remain undigested. Eating food only to make no use of it is simply wasting it. Even worse, food wasted in this way may break down internally into substances that are toxic. Correct food combining not only ensures better nourishment through better digestion, but represents a protective measure against clogging and toxicity.

Adapted from Dr Herbert M. Shelton: *Food Combining . . . Made Easy*,
San Antonio, Texas, 1951.

Many people suffer from acid indigestion, a distended stomach, wind in the intestines (flatulence), allergies to certain foods, obesity, constipation, or any of many other intestinal disorders. It never seems to occur to them that one of the most likely causes of their problem is what they are eating, and especially what they are eating with what. But the food we eat is, of course, closely linked to the traditions and customs of society. Everyone eats bread with cheese, meat with potatoes, rice with beans, a sweet dessert, and perhaps the daily apple or orange to finish off with. Only very recently in circles devoted to dietetics and health, for whom nutrition is the focus of attention, has food combining begun to receive the interest due to it.

Food combining means eating only foods that are suited to each other during any one meal. Some may object that this considerably restricts the choice of food, but it is a fallacious argument. All that is required, when putting together the menu for a meal, is to make a choice that is guided by a knowledge of what the human digestive system is made up of and how it works.

This may seem a strange premise, especially at first. But once familiarity with the rules of food combining has been attained, an individual should never encounter such problems again. The principles become so obvious and so natural that eating correctly no longer requires any mental effort.

The basic idea is to know (and preferably to understand) why some foods can be eaten in combination with each other, and why some cannot. For this it is necessary to have a fair notion of both the physiology and the process of digestion on the one hand, and the chemical composition of foods on the other. Gastroenterologists and nutritionists must have a profound knowledge of such things, of course, but any lay person who is hoping to derive the benefits of healthy nutrition ought to be aware at least of how foods are classified. He or she must know whether a food is high-protein, high-starch, high-fat, high-sugar or high-acid, for example. Some idea of those groups alone should be enough to achieve success. But it will be necessary to master the principles of food combining as quickly as possible, for to interrupt meals in order to carry out calculations over the constitutents of the food being eaten will itself cause indigestion. Sitting at the table, an individual should be able to relax and not worry at all about what he or she is eating: it should be too late by then to be anxious about whether the foods combine.

It is for that very reason that this book presents food combining in a simple and very comprehensible form, with additional notes to help. The main dietary rules are easy to grasp and to remember, and there should be no diminution of appetite. In the early days, before the rules become mere second nature, there will be occasions when serious thought may have to be applied – but that time will soon pass. The diagrams and tables in this book should also prove very helpful.

The theory of food combining is not a recent innovation. It was in fact in 1939 that the American physician Dr Howard Hay (1866–1940) published the first book on the subject. In particular, he pointed out that a combination of high-protein and high-starch foods had appalling effects on the digestion. His compatriot Dr Herbert M. Shelton (1888–1987) then for the decade between 1940 and 1950 carried out intensive research into combinations of specific foods, achieving some significant results and greatly increasing contemporary scientific knowledge of the digestive processes. Shelton discovered that there were combinations which gave rise to excellent, good, problematical, and painful digestion, and he may quite properly be regarded as the true pioneer of food combining. Indeed, he should be counted as one of the most important nutritionists of all time, having even in the 1920s and 1930s published works on aspects of digestion that remain textbooks today.

It is strange that the modern science of dietetics continues to show no interest whatever in food combining. Medical literature is as full now of references to dyspepsia caused by internal fermentation or toxic degradation (the breakdown of ingested food into substances that have some degree of toxicity) as it has ever been. Every family doctor and every hospital intern or house-physician has been asked countless times for advice on dealing with a stomach or intestines distended with wind. In the opinion of most authorities, indigestion results primarily as a consequence of a reduced level of digestive enzymes produced by the pancreas and in the small intestine – which means that digestive discomfort is generally blamed on some form of deficiency in the digestive system, and no account at all is taken of possible deficiencies in the diet.

That Hay and Shelton's nutritional work found little general acceptance is, to be truthful, not entirely incomprehensible. Nutritionists work empirically, judging their results on virtually a statistical basis. Theories are not much to their liking, and even research has to be based on solid evidence. For them it is the results they obtain with actual patients that counts as scientific practice.

Both Hay and Shelton grounded their own work on information contained in a book called *The Operation of the Digestive Organs*, first published in 1902 by the Russian nutritional anatomist Pavlov, who was the first to describe the physiology of the human digestive system in scientific detail. But time and science have moved rapidly on from Pavlov's day, as they have indeed from Hay and Shelton's day: the basic principle formulated by Hay, fundamental also to Shelton's work is now regarded as less than scientific. It was their understanding that starch begins to ferment in the stomach once the salivary enzyme ptyalin is destroyed by gastric juice. How the digestive system works, and the many enzymatic processes that contribute to it, are much better understood now. Had Hay and Shelton's notion been correct, every type of food would be indigestible – acids always surround the food in the stomach, whatever is eaten, and in whatever combination.

It is more than high time for food combining to be studied in depth. The practice of harmonizing specific food types is so important it requires urgent attention. Dr Shelton, with the help of his patients, derived quite a number of food combinations only some of which were inaccurate. It is a pity that even the good ones were not always properly described, a failing that is directly responsible for the regrettable rejection of the whole theory until a few years ago by nutritionists, dieticians and medicine in general.

THE FIVE NUTRIENTS

Food is composed of proteins, fats, carbohydrates, vitamins, minerals, water, and a number of other factors including roughage (dietary fibre), aromatic substances, enzymes, colorants and antioxidants. Only proteins, fats and carbohydrates are subject to digestion, being true nutrients. The process is essentially one of analytical decomposition – chemical breakdown into constituent elements, specifically into these three factors. Whether we eat an apple, a slice of bread, or a steak, digestion breaks the food down into proteins, fats and carbohydrates: protein is broken down further into amino acids, fat into fatty acids, and carbohydrate into simple sugars.

Even if only one type of food is eaten, digestion breaks down all these three nutrients simultaneously. It is completely understandable, then, that opponents of food combining are forever gleefully pointing out that nature herself seems to make for simultaneous digestion of nutrients.

Well, the principle of food combining is quite simple, but other factors also play an important role. The idea that simultaneous digestion of the three nutrients is nature's way will be refuted in due course in this book. But let us adopt a systematic approach.

There are two groups of carbohydrates: sugars and starches. Starches are actually complex sugars, compounds that in their compound form are of no immediate use to the metabolism. They have to be broken down first to double sugars (disaccharides) and then to simple sugars (monosaccharides). Because complex, double, and single sugars occur individually in a large number of foods, however, this book classifies simple and double sugars (including lactose) as 'sugars', and complex sugars as 'starches'. The total number of our nutrient groups is thus enlarged to four.

The fifth and last nutrient group comprises the acids. The acids in food and that affect digestion are free (uncombined) acids, as opposed to bound (or 'conjugate') acids. (Bound acids are released only during metabolism.) Digestion converts the free acids into heat energy, and they are regarded as nutrients accordingly. But they occur only in tiny amounts in foods, and are normally discounted when calculating a food's calorific value.

In food combining, then, the five following nutrient groups represent our principal categories: proteins, fats, sugars, starches, and acids, abbreviated where appropriate to P, F, Su, St and A.

All foods contain these nutrients, and in proportions that are specific to each particular food. The nutrient that is proportionately the greatest in quantity (the dominant nutrient) 'programs' the entire digestive process. To eat different foods at random may result in the presence of more than one dominant nutrient, causing digestive disruption. Reaction between conflicting dominants may cause anything from a mild flush to serious digestive problems involving internal fermentation and gastroenteric poisoning.

Eating only one type of food (a monophagic diet) but in large quantities increases the overall intake of nutrients, although the proportions of the nutrients in relation to each other remain the same. The result would be identical if we were to eat several different foods that are of the same combinatory type. A number of nutrients can be digested during a single meal – on condition that the proportions of nutrients mutually suit each other. These proportions are the key to food combining.

It is obvious (as mentioned above), then, that it is essential to have a good idea of what is the dominant nutrient in every food that is eaten. Only one of the five nutrients can dominate in any one food, and so there are only five possible dominants. The critical factor in compiling a menu for a meal is to do it in such a way as to ensure that there is only one dominant for the whole meal.

Below are several histograms that show the percentage of nutrients in some common foods. In each case, the dominant nutrient is immediately apparent.

beef steak
P: 19 %
F: 4.5 %
Su/St: trace

In beef steak the dominant nutrient is protein, and by a fair margin. The meat does not contain much fat, and there are just traces of the carbohydrates.

avocado
P: 1.9 %
F: 24.0 %
Su/St:0.9 %

Avocado contains mainly fat: fat is evidently the dominant nutrient.

whole-grain rice
P: 7 %
F: 2 %
St: 75 %

The dominant nutrient in whole-grain rice is starch, and the same is true for all cereals and products that include grain, such as bread, waffles and pasta.

banana
P: 1.1 %
F: 0.2 %
Su: 22.0 %

Sugars manifestly dominate this food: the quantity of fats and proteins is almost negligible.

lemon
P: 0.9 %
F: 0.5 %
Su: 8.0 %
A: 4.9 %

Quantitatively, sugars are proportionately the most. But a level of 4.9 per cent acid is very high, and the acid of the fruit has a decisive influence on the digestion – it is acid that is the dominant nutrient.

If we were to eat a beef steak, some whole-grain rice, an avocado, a banana and a lemon during the same meal – actually a very presentable meal in terms of classic nutrition – we would be filling ourselves with five different dominant nutrients. No digestive system is capable of digesting such a meal properly.

A graph showing the dominant nutrients in the five foods.

These examples are clear. But there are some foods in which the dominant nutrient is not so obvious, and that present particular problems of their own: legumes, for example. Leguminous vegetables are remarkable in being dominated by both proteins and starches. This is in fact why they are so difficult to digest. Raw, they are indigestible and potentially toxic because of the fascine acid they contain; cooked, they tend to lie heavy on the stomach and always cause some degree of flatulence. (The herb savory can slightly reduce the flatulence, but not eradicate it altogether.)

The table below shows the percentages of proteins and starches.

Table 1.1
Percentages of nutrients in legumes

	P	F	St	Ratio P:St
white beans	22.0	1.8	47.8	1:2.2
peas	23.0	1.4	60.7	1:3.6
chickpeas	23.5	3.4	50.8	1:2.1
soy(a)beans	36.8	23.5	23.5	1:0.6

In each case there are two 'dominant' nutrients, and in soy(a)beans there are even three. For this reason, legumes are always difficult to digest, whether eaten by themselves or in (a potentially favourable) combination. Although there are methods that can improve matters, digesting legumes requires a lot of energy, so the final metabolic benefit is often not high either.

The protein-starch ratio is more favourable in cereals. But both cereals and legumes are agricultural products that were not part of the diet of early humankind. It was only through the gradual development of agriculture that they were added to the menu, although since then they have dominated human nutrition for more than 10,000 years because of their abundance and their economic value.

As a matter of fact, many ancient civilizations had a keen grasp on which herbs could stimulate and improve digestion. Herbs that were laxatives, or that could moderate diarrhoea, flatulence or colic were much in use. Today's recommendations by newspaper herbalists to try fennel seed, anise or cumin to treat flatulence are but the latest of a tradition that goes back at least as far as the ancient Egyptians, and they probably borrowed the idea from surrounding cultures anyway. Similar traditions of digestive stimulation were current in the pre-Columbian civilizations of South and Central America, albeit with a different selection of herbs. The conclusion is regrettably obvious: humankind has been eating inappropriately for millennia, and has only now begun to learn about food combining.

Table 1.2
Percentages of nutrients in cereal products

	P	F	St	Ratio P:St
millet	10.6	3.9	69.0	1:6.5
maize/corn	9.2	3.8	65.2	1:7
barley	10.6	2.1	57.7	1:5.4
oats	12.6	7.1	61.2	1:4.8
rye	8.7	1.7	53.5	1:6.1
rice	7.4	2.2	74.6	1:10

Starch is the dominant nutrient, but the protein content is relatively high – enough to hinder digestion. The chestnut is a fruit rich in starch, but its protein-starch ratio is different: 3.4 % protein as against 41.2 % starch (ratio 1:12). The greater the P:St ratio, the better the digestibility.

OTHER SUBSTANCES

Books on nutrition quite often suggest that water is significant to the digestive process. A few are also concerned to give roughage (dietary fibre) a role.

Water is indeed a very important constituent of the human body, in which it has a multitude of different functions. Yet water has no direct influence on food combining. Foods rich in water – like fruits, berries, gourds and other vegetables, and of course milk – are easily digestible in comparison with concentrated food sources like nuts, seeds, cereals, cheese and sausages. But the amount of nutrients available for digestion in watery foods is naturally much lower. The brazil nut, for example, has a very favourable protein-fat-sugar-starch ratio, and can be digested without any problems.

One hundred grams (3.5 ounces) of brazil nuts may seem a small quantity of food, but nuts are highly concentrated. The calorific value of 100 grams of brazil nuts is just as much as that of 5 kilograms (11 pounds, fifty times the quantity) of papaya. Food rich in water is in general easier to digest precisely because it contains only a small volume of nutrients. Much less energy is required to release them.

Water has a favourable influence on digestion (the acid-base balance) but not on food combining, although that does not apply to all foods rich in water – after all, meat and fish also have a high water content.

Much the same is true of roughage which, properly defined, is the in-digestible remains of foods that are capable of swelling in the presence of liquids and are sticky and glutinous. Roughage – to which plant fibres such as cellulose, pectin, and a number of other substances belong – is inert in relation to the digestive processes of the stomach and intestines. In the large intestine, however, it swells so as to occupy the complete cross-section of the alimentary canal, and thanks to its stickiness, defecation can be effected easily and smoothly. Important as it may be for this purpose, roughage does not influence food combining. (Some roughage ought always to be present in the diet, nevertheless, to promote defecatory regularity.)

PROCESSED FOODS

The processing of foods may change the proportions of the nutrients within them, sometimes for the better, but sometimes for the worse. Rice has a protein-starch ratio of 1:10. By cooking, a lot of water is absorbed into the rice and a new, more favourable, ratio of 1:12 results.

In bread, on the other hand, the protein-starch ratio remains unchanged. But in starch on its own (as in potato starch, corn starch, rice starch, and so on), the protein-starch ratio is subject to major changes. Such starch is industrially processed as a commercial food ingredient, and the industrial processing generally produces unfavourable ratios. Industrially processed food products have an unfavourable ratio more often than not.

Raw and unprocessed food is generally easier to digest than processed food. But their good properties may have no effect on food combining. Cooked foods may be eaten in combinations that give excellent results and raw foods eaten in combinations that give appalling results, and vice versa. (It is a fallacy that cooked – that is, boiled – food digests more easily than raw food: the food may have so little goodness in it after cooking that there is nothing to be digested, and the food passes virtually straight through untouched by the digestive processes.)

THE ACID-BASE BALANCE

At the beginning of the twentieth century Professor Ragnar Berg (1875–1956) published a study that divided all foods into two basic group-ings, one of 'concentrated foods' and the other of 'unconcentrated foods'. The distinction is readily made because it corresponds fairly well to the difference between high- and low-calorie foods. But for Professor Berg the distinction was not so obvious: the principle behind his classification was whether the foods contained metallic elements or non-metallic elements.

Foods that contain a high proportion of non-metallic elements such as sulphur, phosphorus and chlorine are acid-forming – that is, during the metabolic processes the elements are responsible for the formation of acids. Foods that diminish acidity and are thus effectively alkaline (basic) tend to contain many metallic elements, such as potassium, sodium, magnesium, iron and calcium. Such foods tend also to contain a lot of water but not very much protein. Acid-forming foods, on the other hand, generally contain a fair amount of protein but only a small quantity of water, and the non-metallic elements are ordinarily in the protein.

The acid-base balance has considerable influence on the digestion, and it is thus appropriate to discuss it briefly here. On the pH scale of acidity/alkalinity, human blood varies between 7.3 and 7.5, so it is slightly alkaline (neutral = 7.0). Professor Vincent, the founder of the diagnostic method known as 'Bio-electronics', is of the opinion that for excellent health the blood should ideally be neutral.

To maintain a constant acidity/alkalinity value, the body's acid-base balance makes use of three major mechanisms involving the blood (and substances in it called buffers), the lungs (respiration to remove acidic carbon dioxide) and the kidneys (filtration of acids and alkalis in liquid wastes). The buffers in the blood neutralize excess acids, preventing acidosis. If we were not to rely on these mechanisms at all, we should have to eat a diet of 80–90 per cent alkalizing foods, and only 10–20 per cent acid-forming foods. (In conventional diets, the ratio is more like 55:45.)

Between 80 and 90 per cent of food should be alkalizing, only 10 to 20 per cent acid-forming.

In a conventional diet, the acid–alkali ratio is different: only 55 per cent of the foods are alkalizing, whereas 45 per cent are acid-forming.

The body's acid-base balance thus has considerable influence over the metabolic processes and digestion. As we have seen, foods rich in water are easily digestible. The low proportion of nutrients in relation to the water in such foods corresponds to the ideal ratio between metallic and non-metallic elements.

If we eat too much acid-forming ('concentrated') food, digestion is problematical, even if the foods otherwise combine well.

Meat, fish, cheese, bread, cereals, nuts (and fruit seeds, pits/pips and stones), leguminous vegetables, and so forth, are all acid-forming foods that have a high calorific value.

Fruits, berries, non-leguminous vegetables (including gourds), potatoes (and other tubers and root crops), milk (and non-concentrated milk products like skimmed milk, yoghurt and buttermilk), and so forth, are all alkalizing foods.

Some authorities have presumed that there must also be neutral foods, in which metallic and non-metallic elements work to neutralize each other. Such combinations do not occur in nature, although there are odd foodstuffs like edible oils and household sugar which contain neither metallic nor non-metallic elements. Soft drinks contain only water and sugar to which flavourings and colorants have been added.

The Danish nutritionist Dr Nolfi and others, who were not aware of the theory of food combining but who were intimately concerned with the effects of food on the acid-base balance, derived results that only rarely showed any differences from what might be expected from food combining. The acid-base balance has a critical effect on digestion, on metabolism, and therefore ultimately on overall health.

Interestingly, Dr Hay – unlike Dr Shelton – made a thorough study of this. Yet it was Dr Shelton who recommended the consumption of large quantities of (alkalizing) vegetables when eating preparations of (acid-forming) cereals. He was evidently, if unconsciously, seeking to ensure a good acid-base balance for his patients.

So that no one can misunderstand, it should be emphasized that there is a great difference between acidic food and acid-forming food. Acidic food has an acidic taste – sour, or sour within sweet – whereas acid-forming food is quite another thing and may taste of something else altogether.

It should be stressed in addition that although meat and fish contain a lot of water (perhaps around 75 per cent by volume), they are acid-forming foods. The water content of meat and fish is lower only after it has been smoked or dried. It is not water on which the acid-base balance depends so much as the ratio of metallic to non-metallic elements.

Milk is one of the alkalizing foods, but concentrated milk products (like hard or semi-hard cheese and cottage cheese) are acid-forming foods. The protein content of milk is 3.3 per cent, of cottage cheese between 12 and 18 per cent, and of hard (cheddar, cheshire, emmenthal) and semi-hard (edam, gouda, Port Salut) cheese it is between 25 and 28 per cent.

Cooking food may cause a slight change in the way the food affects the acid-base balance, but it is so small that it may be ignored.

Food combining is extremely important, but is not practised in order to relegate the acid-base balance to relative insignificance. The acid-base balance and food combining represent the focuses of two separate nutritional theories, but both theories support each other.

And indeed there are other dietary factors that have a positive effect on digestion – such as eating slowly, eating little but often, being relaxed during eating, concentrating on the food with sensory anticipation, and so on. Negative factors exist in equal numbers, of course, and include stress and mental tension, emotional upsets, and physical ailments such as gastro-intestinal disorders.

THE NUMBER OF POSSIBLE COMBINATIONS

Anybody who buys a five-digit combination lock relies on the fact that there are countless possible combinations although there are only five digits to make them. A thief has to look for the correct combination among all those possibilities. Fortunately, the possible combinations of foods that harmonize with each other are not so numerous and may be systematized.

There are five nutrients, all of which may be combined as pairs with each other in foods, so there are fifteen possible combinations (discounting combinations that are of the same nutrient, or are merely an inversion of a combination already counted). Combinations of three, four, and five nutrients are also possible. Altogether, then, there is a total of 246 combinations, many of which occur in industrial food products.

Food combining theory reduces the combinations to a total of ten, four of which are good and six of which are bad. They may be schematized in the form of a pentagon. That is not the only way in which the theory may be schematized, but it provides an outline that is fairly easy to memorize and use. To remember the pentagon is always to have on hand all you need to know about food combining. How you can use it is explained later.

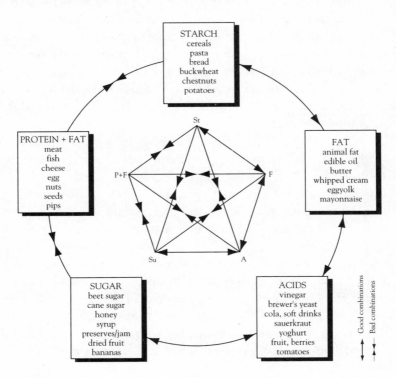

STARCH
cereals
pasta
bread
buckwheat
chestnuts
potatoes

St

PROTEIN + FAT
meat
fish
cheese
egg
nuts
seeds
pips

P+F

FAT
animal fat
edible oil
butter
whipped cream
eggyolk
mayonnaise

F

Su

A

SUGAR
beet sugar
cane sugar
honey
syrup
preserves/jam
dried fruit
bananas

ACIDS
vinegar
brewer's yeast
cola, soft drinks
sauerkraut
yoghurt
fruit, berries
tomatoes

Good combinations
Bad combinations

Reading the books by the various cookery experts, gastronomes and TV cuisine artistes, it is amazing how often the rules of food combining are flouted.

THE CHOICE OF FOOD

Before looking at the classification of foods and the physiology of human digestion, it is advisable to look at the choice of food – that is, at how to choose foods that are in harmony with the anatomy and functional physiology of the digestive system.

It is notable that in the animal world each species has its own eating pattern. Biologists distinguish between carnivores (meat-eaters), herbivores (plant-eaters), granivores (seed- and grain-eaters) and fructivores (fruit-eaters). The digestive system of a carnivore is completely different from that of a herbivore: a dog, fox, or cat digests in a manner totally different from a cow, rabbit, or goat. Granivorous creatures like the chicken and other gallinaceous birds have a beak, a crop, a glandular stomach, a muscular stomach, a pancreas with three outlet ducts, and lengthy intestines (guts) with tiny follicles (cavities). Their digestive system is entirely focused on the processing of starch in grains and seeds. Primates are mostly fruit-eaters, surviving by consuming berries and nuts: their very specific digestive system is able to derive surprising amounts of energy from small quantities of food.

Humankind is supposed to be omnivorous, eating everything and not caring two hoots about the choice of food. That choice is determined, in advanced countries at least, by advertising, price, taste, fashion, and culinary expertise, among other factors.

The health of human beings has never been uniformly excellent, as we have already seen. The history of gastric ailments to a great extent mirrors the history of agriculture. To be more accurate, it could be said that the history of indigestion runs parallel with the history of inappropriate food combining. Humans just pile the food all together and swallow it down with no thought for their digestive systems; naturally enough the results are painful and debilitating, and people remain susceptible to all kinds of disease.

It is generally agreed by palaeontologists that humans are by nature herbivorous – plant-eaters – but became omnivorous by teaching themselves to eat other things, almost like learning a skill. So today we eat meat, fish, cereals, milk, fruit and nuts in addition to vegetables. And most of us eat them all at once. Another consequence is that, despite the millennia of evolution and cultural development, humans have no single characteristic that places them well and truly among the carnivores, the herbivores or the granivores. To eat meat, humans often require a tooth-pick: unlike a dog's teeth, human teeth are rather too close together for comfortable meat-eating. Humans cannot digest grass at all – indeed, many people have severe problems digesting raw vegetables. And in spite of 10,000 years of agriculture during which grains and cereals have formed a predominant part of the diet, humans still do not have a beak, a crop, or a dual stomach.

What we do have is a dual problem: we eat foods that are not attuned to our digestive systems, and most of us have no idea how to combine foods properly.

This book is of course concerned to rectify that last problem. It was Dr Shelton's dictum that all the foods we eat should be combined in a useful way. The theory of food combining can be applied to all eating patterns. It is in the interest of every single person to combine foods appropriately, whether he or she is a conventional meat-and-fish eater or a vegetarian. The more natural the eating pattern that one adopts, the easier it is to combine food harmoniously. A fruit-eater (who may eat melons and nuts as well as fruits and berries) gains little from food combining. On the other hand, people with the conventional eating patterns can benefit most from food combining.

The fact that food combining can be applied to all eating patterns is its one great advantage: it is not just for health freaks and vegetarians, and certainly not just for people who are weak or ill, but for everyone.

THE EFFECTS OF FOOD COMBINING

Someone who really makes an effort with food combining should achieve constantly perfect digestion. There is no need to resort to forceful persuasion on the subject: it should be enough to test the combinations for oneself. After a meal consisting of appropriately combined foods one should leave the table without feeling bloated or heavy, without any sensation of fatigue, but feeling satisfied while at the same time having nothing to remind one that one has in fact just eaten. As long as one's digestive processes are operating at an optimum, one's body weight will automatically regulate itself, and weight will be gained or lost until the ideal weight is attained. Acid indigestion, feeling bloated, and flatulence are gone forever. There is a good chance too that a person who has been suffering from a food allergy will discover that he or she is no longer allergic: many food allergies result from the presence of toxic substances in the intestines that are there only because of inappropriate food combining. Residues of undigested proteins can be particularly toxic, for example. Pressed against the intestinal wall, they may pass through into the bloodstream and cause a systemic allergic reaction.

The normal intestinal bacteria (the flora) depend for their life and function on the food that is ingested. Occasionally, certain bacteria increase rapidly and disproportionately, disrupting the floral balance. If the food residues that cause this originate from starch, fermentation occurs, causing the formation of lactic acid and short-chain fatty acids. The fatty acids then irritate the intestinal wall, sensitizing it in a way that quite frequently leads to diarrhoea.

Disruption of the normal floral balance can have even more serious consequences if the causative factor is protein residues. Undigested proteins form peptides and amino acids that may be converted into amines by the unusually disproportionate intestinal flora, and amines are both unpleasantly pungent and toxic. Whereas odourless intestinal gas caused by fermentation is not especially serious, pungent intestinal gas can be dangerous. The protein residues damage the intestinal wall in such a way as to cause it to secrete fluid and protein as nourishment for the intestinal flora. The amines may eventually pass through the intestinal wall and travel on in the bloodstream all the way up to the brain.

Diarrhoea due to the presence of toxic substances in the intestine is usually the result of a combination of protein and starch.

A number of disorders are caused primarily by dysfunction of the intestines. In all too many people, the large intestine is a disgustingly smelly duct at all times partly clogged with faeces. Constipation, which is extremely common, can lead eventually to acidosis and even poisoning of the tissues, and the consequent contamination of adjacent organs. The majority of inhabitants in advanced countries have intestines that are to some degree subject to acidosis and poisoning. Medication does not help much – only good food combining can really improve the condition. In this way, in particular, food combining could be of supreme importance.

Using appropriate combinations of foods is the way to perfect digestion, through which the body purifies itself by eliminating toxic substances and by not allowing any more of them to be produced. The floral balance in the intestines is restored, as is the regularity of daily bowel movements. A clean intestine means less activity by the liver and potential relief to surface tissues. Sometimes even sleeping disorders can be traced to the effects of poorly functioning intestines, and food combining may therefore contribute to a good night's sleep after years of insomnia.

Obesity should disappear, as should any feeling of bloating or distension in the stomach and intestines, bringing a sense of wellbeing and even improving self-confidence in one's appearance.

Thousands of people who applied these simple dietary rules were amazed that food combining was able to change their lives so radically and so immediately. Basic health may certainly be said to depend on combining appropriate foods, although not all health problems can be solved so easily. Yet recovery from just about any ailment or disorder can be assisted through the use of food combining.

To do justice to food combining, particular attention must be paid to maintaining a good acid-base balance, to the correct choice of foods, and to moderation in the quantity of what we eat and drink.

CHAPTER 2

THE CLASSIFICATION OF FOODS

Conventional eating habits violate all the rules of food combining. Most people seem quite content to put up with years of pain, hardship, and frequent attacks of disease; only a very few are prepared to rethink their eating strategy with any genuine consideration. Whenever the idea of food combining surfaces, people usually declare that as far as the bad combinations are concerned, they regularly swallow them down and feel none the worse at all afterwards. At that rate, life and death, health and sickness are merely incidental to them. But unfortunately they are encouraged in this attitude by their medical advisers.

For many years I have been prescribing a diet for both the healthy and the sick, for both the weak and the strong, the old and the young. And in all this time it has ever been the case that a conversion to good food combining is followed by an immediate improvement in overall health.

Adapted from Dr Herbert M. Shelton: *Food Combining . . . Made Easy*,
San Antonio, Texas, 1951.

To apply beneficial combinations of food – and to avoid potentially disastrous ones – the dominant nutrient of every food to be eaten must be known. There are up to five nutrients in any food. In most, only one is dominant. When two or three vie for dominance, the food is not easily digestible even if eaten by itself (as is the case with legumes). Combining such a food with others usually makes it even more difficult to digest.

Foods are classified in five groups, each with subdivisions.

1. PROTEINS

Proteins are polymers that consist of compounds of twenty amino acids. Unlike carbohydrates or fats, proteins contain a very large number of constituent elements. The number of different proteins that can be built up from amino acids is quite high. We cannot produce the eight 'essential' amino acids by ourselves, however: they must be supplied in the food we eat. The usefulness of protein derived from food is thus determined by the presence of these eight essential amino acids.

The digestion of protein occurs by means of enzymes produced in the stomach, the pancreas and the wall of the small intestine. Following protein digestion there are always waste products or acids, for the process is naturally difficult. The proteins thus require particular attention in relation to food combining.

At this point suffice to say that three types of protein are distinguishable: animal protein, lactoprotein, and vegetable protein. In the next chapter it is shown that each of these types of protein has its own process in human digestion (which is why it is important to list the types from the beginning).

For many years it was thought that animal protein was vital to life, an opinion that was quite understandable in that vegetable protein and lacto-protein contain none of the essential amino acids that animal protein does.

Mind you, the debate still continues over the daily requirement of protein. For too long the basis of consideration was body weight. Now we know that other factors are of much more importance. Heat changes the properties of a protein by altering its structure, destroying the protective jacket of water around the protein molecule. It is important for us to combine proteins in the correct way in order to improve our digestion of them, which is already problematical.

The actual need for protein depends both on digestion and on the quality of the protein: good food combining can drastically reduce the need for protein, thereby also reducing the waste products. This is a measure of how important food combining can be in relation to high-protein food.

In nature, protein occurs only in the presence of fat. In meat and fish, the proportions of protein and fat are relatively quite different, with protein predominant by far. In concentrated milk products like (hard and semi-hard) cheese, the proportions are closer to each other. And in nuts (and fruit seeds, pits/pips and stones) the fat content usually exceeds the protein content. Nonetheless, all of these are rich in protein. The fat content can be increased by cooking: fish dishes can be cooked in oil, for example. Similarly, the fat content can be reduced by using low-fat milk products or lean meat, and so on.

To be considered high-protein, a food must consist of at least 10 per cent protein. All meat and fish contain a lot of protein, including types of meat and fish that are relatively fatty. Exceptions are cod liver (6 per cent), bacon (4.1 per cent) and kidney lard (1.2 per cent), which are not so much high-protein foods as high-fat foods.

In terms of lactoprotein, only milk products in concentrated form are regarded as high-protein. For convenience, however, eggs are also classified within the lactoprotein group.

Another exception, but in terms of vegetable high-protein foods, is the coconut. It is actually a low-protein nut, containing only 4.2 per cent protein. Coconut flakes contain 5.6 per cent protein and 62 per cent fat – so it is a high-fat foodstuff.

Dried mushrooms are rich in proteins, but the water that is added in cooking them reduces the protein content. The same is true of cocoa powder, which is also high-protein although when it is processed into the form of chocolate or chocolate milk the protein content comes no higher than 10 per cent.

The tables below present an accurate guide to the quantities of protein contained in specific foods that are regarded as high-protein.

Animal protein

veal	22.0 %
beef	21.3 %
pork	21.1 %
rabbit	20.9 %
chicken	20.6 %
horse meat	20.6 %
lamb/mutton	20.4 %
dried fish	20–79 %
game	20–22 %
goat meat	19.5 %
fish products	16–21 %
poultry	15–24 %
freshwater fish	15–20 %
saltwater fish	15–19 %
meat products	11–29 %
crustaceans	9–18.6 %

Lactoprotein

powdered egg yolk	46.2 %
powdered buttermilk	38.6 %
powdered skimmed milk	35.3 %

powdered egg white	31.1 %
powdered whole milk	25.5 %
egg yolk	16.1 %
chicken's egg	12.9 %
cottage cheese	11–13 %
egg white	10.9 %
hard/semi-hard cheese	9.2–32.2 %

Vegetable protein

dried brewer's yeast	48.0 %
peanut butter	47.8 %
soya flour	43.4 %
rye germ	42.0 %
soy(a)beans	36.8 %
wheatgerm	28.0 %
peanuts	26.0 %
seeds	20–36 %
dried legumes	19–23.9 %
pips	13–27 %
nuts	13–19 %
baker's yeast	1.1 %

2. FATS

Fats, or lipids, include most substances that are insoluble in water and that are present in all cells. Most foods contain some.

In foods, they are almost always to be found together with protein. To absorb fats from ingested food, to digest them, and to metabolize concentrated forms, the body makes use of two indispensable fluids: bile (occasionally known as gall) and pancreatic juice. The digestion of fats begins as late as in the duodenum, and is comparatively separate from the rest of the digestive process. Only people who suffer from dysfunction of the gall-bladder (which secretes bile) or from a diseased liver tend to have any problem in digesting fats.

Fat combines readily with starch, a combination that retards the activity of the stomach – a property that in turn can prove useful in relation to digesting some combinations of foods but may cause difficulties in relation to others.

Because fat and protein are ordinarily together in foods, it is necessary always to check which of them is the dominant nutrient in any one food. Protein tends to dominate combinations of food, whereas fats tend to be comparatively subordinate. But consuming a large quantity of fatty food in which the protein proportion is higher than 10 per cent runs the risk of creating a poor combination if the food is eaten together with starchy foods.

Egg yolk contains 16.1 per cent protein and 32 per cent fat. In theory, protein should be the dominant nutrient because the protein content is higher than 10 per cent, although the fat content is double that of the protein by volume. In practice, it is rather different. Egg yolk is always used in small amounts. One egg yolk contains about 3 grams (0.1 ounces) of protein and 6 grams (0.2 ounces) of fat. If one egg yolk is incorporated in a meal, the effect is virtually negligible.

Just as proteins are grouped according to whether they are animal-, vegetable- or milk-based, so there are animal, vegetable and milk fats. In connection with food combining there is no need to make a further distinction between saturated, unsaturated and polyunsaturated fatty acids.

Animal fat

cod liver oil	99.9 %
melted lard	99.7 %
beef fat/dripping	96.5 %
kidney lard	94.4 %
bacon	65.0 %

Milk fats

butter	83.2 %
whipped cream (40%)	40.0 %
egg yolk	32.0 %
whipped cream (10%)	10.0 %

Vegetable fats

corn oil	99.9 %
safflower oil	99.9 %
soya oil	99.9 %

palm oil	99.8 %
sunflower oil	99.8 %
cottonseed oil	99.7 %
olive oil	99.6 %
linseed oil	99.5 %
sesame oil	99.5 %
peanut oil	99.4 %
walnut oil	91.5 %
coconut oil	90.0 %
mayonnaise	80.0 %
margarine (all kinds)	80.0 %
coconut flakes	62.0 %
avocado	24.0 %
black olives	17.0 %
green olives	13.3 %

3. SUGARS

Although sugars and starches are all carbohydrates, they behave very differently in combination with other foods – which is why they are treated separately here. This section thus concerns foods rich in sugars, and in which sugars represent the dominant nutrient.

Sugars are subdivided into milk sugars and vegetable sugars. Honey is a vegetable product despite being produced through the agency of bees. Some people refuse to eat honey on ethical grounds but, purely from a nutritional point of view, it is an excellent food.

A number of fruits have a sugar content of more than 12 per cent, and in these fruits sugar is the dominant nutrient, although a different grouping is made in the section on acids: some fruits that are rich in sugar also contain large amounts of acid.

Milk sugars have a generally low value: they are included really only for interest. Milk is a nutritious food but it is difficult to combine with other foods.

Milk sugar (lactose)

mother's milk	7.1 %
horse's milk	6.2 %
cow's milk	4.8 %

goat's milk	4.8 %
sheep's milk	4.7 %

Vegetable sugar

industrial sugar	100 %
brown cane sugar	98 %
honey	91 %
sweets	84–97 %
soft drinks	82 %
preserves	80 %
jam	63 %
apple syrup	60 %
maple syrup	60 %
fruit cordial	57 %
chocolate	54 %

Fruits rich in sugar

dried fruit	55 %
sweetened canned fruit	60 %
fruit concentrate	57 %

banana	23.0 %
wild bilberry	19.6 %
rose-hip	19.3 %
cultivated bilberry	19.0 %
grape juice	17.1 %
lychee	17.0 %
grape	16.8 %
mirabelle plum	15.5 %
greengage	13.5 %
passion fruit	13.4 %
fresh fig	12.9 %
mango	12.8 %
sweet cherry	12.7 %
nectarine	12.4 %
honeydew melon	12.0 %
redcurrant juice	12.0 %

cactus fig	12.0 %
plum	11.9 %
pomegranate	11.6 %

4. STARCH

Starch belongs to the group of polysaccharides or complex sugars: it is the most important form in which saccharides (sugars) are found in plant cells. It is present in large quantities in the seeds particularly of grasses like buckwheat and in chestnuts, carrots, tubers, root crops, stalks, and sometimes in fruits and leaves.

Many of the starch-rich parts of plants are important sources of nourishment for humans and animals, and are therefore of major economic significance. These include potatoes, wheat, maize/corn, rice, oats, barley, rye, buckwheat, leguminous vegetables, soya, cassava (from which tapioca is derived), arrowroot, and sago (from the pith of a variety of palm).

Starch is important to conventional nutrition. A substantial proportion of all the world's agricultural production for human or animal consumption consists of starchy foods.

Most books on nutrition emphasize the importance of starch as a source of energy. From an economic viewpoint this makes good enough sense, but from a purely nutritional angle differing opinions are beginning to make themselves heard. An analysis of the results of food combining leads directly to the conclusion that foods rich in starch are extremely difficult to combine with other foods, and indeed all such combinations tend to cause a plethora of digestive problems.

Because starch is a ubiquitous ingredient in food, however, a lot of attention must be devoted to it at this point.

Starch is present exclusively in vegetable foods, although there is a type of animal starch called glycogen. Glycogen is a sort of precursor of glucose in the body, stored in organs such as the liver, the heart and the tongue. As a constituent in food, the amount is so small that it can be ignored in relation to food combining.

Although the different kinds of starch combine freely, the lists below distinguish between the various farinaceous foods, so providing a better insight into their great variety.

Cereal starch

Grains

white rice	78 %
whole-grain rice	75 %
millet	69 %
maize/corn	65 %
oats	61 %
wheat	60 %
barley	58 %
rye	54 %

Flour

rice flour	79 %
cornflakes	74 %
barley flour	72 %
wheat flour	72 %
popcorn	68 %
cornflour	65 %
rye flour	65 %
oatmeal	61 %

Bread

crispbread	66 %
rusk	61 %
wholemeal rusk	58 %
white bread	48 %
rye bread	45 %
puff pastry	37 %

Pasta

spaghetti	75 %
noodles	65 %
wholewheat noodles	64 %

Seeds

buckwheat	71 %
buckwheat flour	71 %
chestnut	41 %

Individual starches

corn starch	86 %
rice starch	85 %
tapioca starch	85 %
potato starch	83 %
wheat starch	83 %

Vegetables rich in starch

potato crisps/chips	53.0 %
potato chips/fries	35.0 %
potato croquette	20.0 %
raw potato	15.4 %
boiled potato	14.0 %
horseradish	11.7 %
ginger	11.0 %
mashed potato	11.0 %

Vegetables low in starch

garlic	6.0 %
pumpkin	5.0 %
grean beans (pods)	5.0 %
winter radish	4.1 %
Jerusalem artichoke	4.0 % (inulin, a starch substitute)
kohlrabi	4.0 %
chicory	3.0 %
asparagus	2.0 %
Chinese leaves/cabbage	2.0 %
mushrooms	1.0 %
endive	1.0 %
blanched celery	1.0 %
green pepper	1.0 %
red pepper	1.0 %
parsley	1.0 %
radish	1.0 %
spinach	1.0 %
parsnip	0.5 %
celeriac	0.4 %

– values lower than 4 per cent can be disregarded

Starch-free vegetables and herbs
  onion
  chervil
  cucumber
  gherkin
  swede
  purslane
  turnip
  rhubarb
  red cabbage
  white cabbage
  salsify
  lettuce
  Brussels sprouts
  tomatoes
  garden cress
  lamb's lettuce
  fennel
  watercress
  aubergine/eggplant
  courgette
  cauliflower
  broccoli
  carrots
  chives
  dandelion
  nettle
  leek
  shallot
  finocchio/Florence fennel
  carrot tops
  garden sorrel

5. ACIDS

This section is concerned with those foods in which acids have an effect on food combining. The acids involved are free acids (see Chapter One: The Acid–Base Balance).

A distinction is made between the degree of acidity (the pH value) and the acid content, which is the constituent proportion of acids expressed as a percentage by volume. The more acids there are, the lower is the pH value; the less acid there is, the higher the pH value. These are the acids that can damage the salivary enzyme ptyalin and slow down the production of gastric juice – but they usually have a corresponding number of beneficial properties too.

The lists below distinguish between individual acids, acidic drinks, lactic acid products, and acids in fruits. Apart from tomatoes, vegetables contain few acids. Their degree of acidity varies between pH 5 and pH 6.6.

Individual acids by pH value

vinegar	1.8
wine vinegar	2.2
cider vinegar	2.4
brewer's yeast	4.5

Acidic drinks

cola	1.9
wine	2.1
fizzy lemonade	2.5
bitter lemon	2.6
tonic water	2.6
fizzy orangeade	2.7
beer/lager	2.9
port	3.2
fizzy mineral water	4.0
instant coffee	4.9
tea brewed properly	5.4

Lactic acid products

liquid with cocktail onions	2.7
vegetables containing lactic acid	3.2
sauerkraut	3.4
liquid with sweet-sour gherkins	3.7

live organic yoghurt	3.9
live yoghurt	4.0

Acids in fruits

Mildly acidic fruits (acid as % volume)

papaya	0.20–0.50
pear	0.20–0.50
cherry	0.20–0.60
mango	0.20–1.20
pomegranate	0.40–1.00
apple	0.40–1.20
banana	0.45
plum	0.50
strawberry	0.50
grape	0.70
peach	0.70
orange	0.80
pineapple	0.80
guava	0.80
sweet sloe	0.80
quince	0.95
(pH values 3.6–3.9)	

Semi-acidic fruits

elderberry	1.20
apricot	1.30
raspberry	1.30
bilberry	1.30
kiwi fruit	1.60
fairly sharp orange	1.60
fairly sharp grape	1.60
gooseberry	1.60
blackberry	1.80
morello cherry	1.80
rowan berry	2.00
grapefruit	2.10
redcurrant	2.50
cowberry	2.60
(pH values 3.0–3.5)	

Acidic fruits

sour cherry	3.00
rose-hip	3.10
whitecurrant	3.10
whitebeam	3.30
blackcurrant	3.30
passion fruit	3.40
sour sloe	3.50
cranberry	3.80
sea-buckthorn	3.80
lemon	4.90
(pH values 2.0–2.9)	

CHAPTER 3

THE DIGESTION

Every year millions of dollars are spent on medicinal drugs that can provide only temporary relief from the discomfort and misery caused by the decomposition of food in the stomach and intestines.

The people of the United States consume veritable cartloads of preparations aimed at neutralizing acid, eliminating intestinal gas, easing pain, and even relieving headaches caused by overstimulation of the stomach. Hormonal substances and enzymes like pepsin are used to aid digestion. And yet it is the pain and distress that is considered the normal condition, and the rare anxiety-free state is ironically seen as abnormal.

Feeling happy and resting easy are the hallmarks of good health; pain and discomfort are not. Normal digestion cannot be equated with any sign or symptom of disorder.

Adapted from Dr Herbert M. Shelton: *Food Combining . . . Made Easy*,
San Antonio, Texas, 1951.

The point of food combining is to ensure normal and easy digestion after eating several foods during one meal. Just like animals today, early humans ate only one kind of food per meal.

It is sometimes claimed that cows munch more than one type of grass, or grass containing other plants, at the same time. Certainly the flourishing natural meadows, especially alpine meadows, contain a rich variety of vegetation, but for all that, the variety is in fact limited to either gramineous or herbaceous plants. And each cow is scrupulously fastidious in its selection of what it eats – all herbivores are equally careful – steering well clear of buttercups, for example, or any grass that has grown up through a patch of dung. In savanna regions, most animals eat only certain grasses and leave the rest. By instinct, animals know what to eat, and what food does or does not go together.

Humans are now supposedly civilized. They cultivate crops to eat, and go to elaborate lengths to prepare their food. Some commentators see an

33

improvement in this, but humans cannot change their evolutionary nature quite so easily. They are still bound by a number of physiological laws, and especially those relating to digestion. It should not be forgotten that the human digestive system has actually changed very little since prehistoric times. The modern food industry may come up with delicious food products prepared in the most appetizing way, but those products may be scarcely digestible because no one has thought to take human digestive physiology into consideration. At the same time, people cannot be expected to eat nothing but natural foods such as fruits and nuts.

Mind you, some people do eat only fruits and nuts, and they have little need of food combining. Their eating pattern is so simple, and their choice of foods so restricted, that it is virtually impossible for them to transgress the rules of food combining.

The average person, however, and anyone who has some respect for their health, prefers a varied diet. Such a person does not have to live a secluded life surrounded by rules that few others adhere to: eating can be a highly social activity. Food should never dominate one's lifestyle, never become more than simply a part of life.

The main theme of this book is food combining, and it is specifically in that connection that this chapter looks at digestion and the human digestive system. The anatomy and physiology of the digestive system are covered relatively cursorily except where they impinge on aspects related to food combining, when all necessary information is provided. This is essential to an understanding of how food combining works and what benefits it can impart.

THE DIGESTIVE SYSTEM

The digestive system may be considered to comprise the alimentary canal, the long tract that begins at the mouth and ends at the anus. Its overall length is usually between 7 and 8 metres (23–26 feet). The mechanism that does the digesting is a process on the inner surface of parts of the canal, but its overall surface area is a staggering 400 square metres (475 square yards). Such an enormous surface area is made possible by the complex structure of the stomach and intestinal wall. Just as the plants in a field obtain their nourishment from the ground, the human body gets its nourishment from the surface of the digestive system. The larger the surface, the better the nutrients can be absorbed.

The process of digestion is one of decomposition: the breaking down of many substances into their basic constituents. An apple, for example, is made up of water, protein, fat, carbohydrates, vitamins, minerals, fruit acids, colouring, flavouring, and so on. Digestion releases all these substances (many of which are themselves compounds) to be used as best they may for nourishment. Of these released substances, those that do not become building-blocks of tissue growth contribute to the process of metabolism by being converted to energy.

Digestion takes place through the agency of enzymes, catalysts that promote biochemical processes. Their effect depends on the degree of acidity (the pH value) present in the environment in which they are active. If the degree of acidity changes rapidly or markedly, their activity comes to a halt.

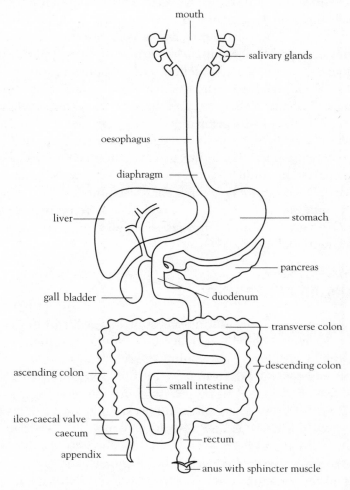

A schematic representation of the digestive tract.

The digestive system begins at the mouth, in which the salivary glands and the tongue are located. Between the mouth and the stomach extends the tubular passage called the oesophagus. The stomach is a J-shaped sac in which food is mixed with gastric juice and churned around and thoroughly kneaded by muscles in the stomach wall. Bile, which emulsifies fats, is secreted by the gallbladder into the duodenum, in many respects the centre of the digestive process. The pancreas likewise produces three fluids that digest fats, carbohydrates and protein. Digestion continues in the small intestine, from which the elements broken down are absorbed through the intestinal wall, leaving only waste materials and water to go further. The absorbed nutrients are taken by the bloodstream to the liver, where many further processes take place. From the small intestine, the intestinal contents are fed gradually into the caecum through the ileo-caecal valve, and on to the large intestine. The function of the large intestine is only nominally digestive but is critical to the physical sensation of digestion as experienced by the individual, and to the completion of the whole endeavour. Water and other fluids are removed from the waste matter, the faeces are formed and compacted, and they are finally excreted through the rectum and anus.

Within the length of this canal many digestive processes take place. If our diet consisted of only one type of food, we should never experience any problems with digestion. But eating several different types of food at the same time makes digestion more difficult – unless we take into account which foods can and cannot be combined. Meals should be compiled so that the natural processes of digestion can go ahead in the optimal fashion, and this is made entirely possible through the combining of foods that are harmonious with each other.

THE PHYSIOLOGY OF DIGESTION

Tracing the processes of digestion means studying each part of the digestive system in turn, including wherever necessary some anatomical description and detail. But even at its very beginning, the complexities inherent in digestion become obvious: the lips form the transition between two very different and highly sensitive areas of tissue: the skin and the mucous membrane of the mouth. The digestive system does not exist on its own but is connected intimately with the nervous and vascular systems. It is regulated by the hypothalamus, a delicate cherry-sized area of the forebrain behind the eyes.

But the digestive system is even more elaborate and sensitive. All the senses and all the emotions can affect the function of the digestive system.

This is important because digestive problems can be caused by any of a multitude of physical and mental aspects, including emotional disorders, anxiety and stress. The careful practice of food combining is not enough on its own: our disposition, the way we obtain food, and what food means to us are just as important. A person who eats when not hungry will digest badly. A person who sits down at the table when not having expected to and looked forward to it, or who eats the meal in a mood of anger, fear or exasperation, will not benefit even from well-chosen combinations of foods. Humans do not eat with their mouths only, but with their eyes, noses, and with their whole beings. That is absolutely crucial to understand.

The Mouth

The mouth surrounds the oral cavity – the space confined by the lips, cheeks and jaws – and is lined with epithelial cells in the form of mucous membrane. Structures in the mouth comprise the teeth and gums, the soft and hard palates, and the tongue (and the sublingual tissues). Three pairs of salivary glands produce saliva to lubricate the mouth. And predominantly on the tongue are the taste-buds, some 10,000 of them in four different types spread over eight major areas, by means of which all flavours are discerned.

The function of the teeth is to crush food: incisors cut and slice food into pieces; molars grind food into pulp; and the canine teeth are used both to hold food steady as the incisors bite into it, and to reduce hard, large pieces of food to smaller, more manageable chunks. Only when eating natural types of food in a natural manner – as we may when eating apples, berries and raw carrots, for example – do we make complete use of our teeth. Most of the time the food we eat has already been chopped into small pieces, and cooked or baked in the kitchen.

In a way, the mouth corresponds to a personal kitchen. It is amazing just how much the kitchen has, conversely, taken over the duties of the mouth. One consequence of the food's having been chopped smaller or softened beforehand is that we run the perennial risk of not producing enough saliva: the food may be swallowed too quickly for saliva to come into play.

Saliva has not one but at least two effects on food. It is the first element of the digestive process, acting on starch and protein even before the food is swallowed. And it forms a wrapping around the food, a protective and lubricating layer that facilitates swallowing and the subsequent passage down to the stomach. This wrapping, moreover, kills inimical bacteria.

The composition of saliva is not uniformly the same but depends on the site of secretion and the speed with which it is produced. One important constituent is alpha-amylase ptyalin, an enzyme capable of breaking down starch, a process that thus begins as early as in the mouth. Such a digestive effect on food even before it is swallowed is known as predigestion.

Saliva is produced initially by reflex action, prompted by the stimuli of the smell and taste of food. Then the presence of the food in contact with the mucous membrane of the mouth together with the chewing movements of the lower jaw elicit further secretion of saliva.

The production of saliva is also influenced by the type of food that is taken into the mouth. Foods rich in starch (such as bread, potatoes or chestnuts) elicit large amounts of saliva, whereas high-protein foods generate lesser quantities. A chestnut taken into the mouth has to be chewed for a long time, and an abundance of saliva is produced; a hazel nut or an almond simply does not have the same effect. To cut short the time spent chewing, humans took to roasting chestnuts or toasting bread. But by heating, the starch is destroyed. Without the starch, or at least the digestible starch, the chestnuts might as well be hazel nuts or almonds, and only a lesser amount of saliva is produced accordingly.

Every day, our mouths produce between 1 and 1.5 litres (about 2 pints) of saliva. Among other constituents it contains calcium salts and phosphates which between them regulate the degree of acidity (the pH) of the saliva, a property that is of great importance to the overall function of ptyalin. Researchers of former decades, like the good doctors Hay and Shelton, reckoned that ptyalin was only active in an alkaline environment. We now know better. Ptyalin functions best in an environment that is between neutral and slightly acid, optimally between pH values of 7 and 5.5. In any case, there are no foods that are neutral or alkaline as such.

Food that is rich in starch should be combined only with foods that do not reduce the pH value in the mouth. Acid with starch is a bad combination: foods that are excessively acidic nullify the function of the ptyalin.

The Stomach

The human stomach has a very special shape. Not very large, its outer wall is made up of layers of muscle. It too has more than one function. But the stomach is primarily where food descending from the mouth, chewed and bathed in saliva, is mixed with gastric juice. How acidic that gastric juice is depends upon the type of food: large amounts of high-protein food lead to a high degree of acidity (a low pH value).

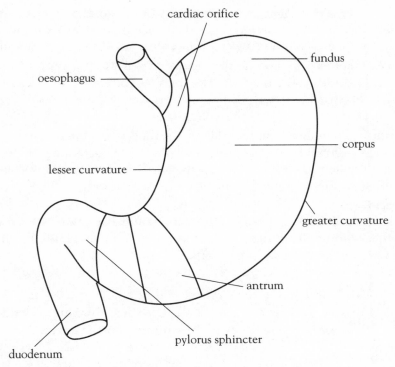

The parts and technical terms of the human stomach.

No matter what kind of food is eaten, the contents of the stomach are always bathed in acid. The acids produced by and in the stomach have three major purposes: first to rid the food of inimical bacteria; second to stabilize the sugars released under the influence of the salivary enzyme or eaten directly; and third to break down protein. This last function is carried out by the enzyme pepsin, which can only work in an acidic environment.

The gastric juice in the stomach of an infant is less acidic: milk fat undergoes an initial digestive phase in the stomach through the agency of the enzyme lipase. The phase is of only minor significance in adults.

Gastric Juice

Some 3 litres (5 or 6 pints) of gastric juice are secreted by the stomach every day. The most important constituents in it are the enzyme that breaks down protein (pepsin, in all its varieties), hydrochloric acid (HCl), and mucus (mucin).

39

There are altogether eight different pepsins that are created when parts of the molecule of the substances that are their precursor states (pepsinogens) are split off; they have a pH value of less than 6. By itself, hydrochloric acid would ensure a pH value for the gastric juice of around 1. It is increased to an overall value of between 2 and 4 by the buffer effect of the pulpy food-and-acid mixture to which the stomach contents are reduced, called chyme. Pepsins work best at these acidity values.

The mucous membrane on the walls of the fundus and the corpus contain primary cells, secondary cells, and surface cells. Pepsinogens are produced in the primary cells, hydrochloric acid in the surface cells, and the secondary cells secrete mucus which protects the stomach wall against the hydrochloric acid.

Digestive fluids are produced in the stomach and elsewhere as a result of any of three stimuli: the influence of the senses and the mind, local stomach mechanisms, and intestinal mechanisms.

The senses and the mind. Seeing, tasting, and/or smelling food causes the secretion of gastric juice as a reflex action. Even just thinking of food can start it off. Emotions strongly influence the stimulation, or the inhibition, of gastric juice secretion. Tension and aggression cause more gastric juice to be produced, and can lead over time to a stomach ulcer as the acidic juice attacks the stomach wall. Fear, on the other hand, retards the production of gastric juice, the absence of which can make digestion very difficult.

Stomach mechanisms. When the chyme arrives in the lower areas of the stomach, in particular the antrum, the hormone gastrin is released into the bloodstream. It circulates back up to the higher parts of the stomach, where it causes further secretion of gastric juice. This is part of the mechanism by which the stomach keeps track of exactly where the food is and what stage of digestion it has reached, secreting gastric juice as required.

Intestinal mechanisms. Gastrin is released into the circulation not only in the antrum of the stomach, but outside the stomach altogether, in the first part of the intestine, the duodenum. It is there too that the hormone secretin and a specific peptide are released into the bloodstream, and together have the effect of slowing down the secretion of gastric juice, negating the action of the juice-stimulating gastrin. The contrasting actions of gastrin and secretin thus act as another regulatory mechanism.

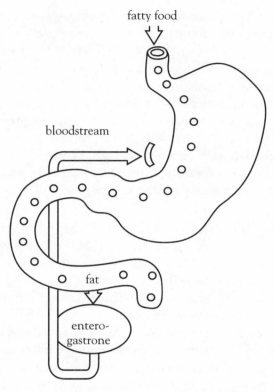

fatty food

bloodstream

fat

entero-
gastrone

When fat reaches the duodenum, the hormone enterogastrone is released into the bloodstream. Travelling back up to the stomach, the hormone there slows down the secretion of gastric juice and the digestive movements of the stomach wall.

The action of the stomach. As the stomach gradually fills, which occurs in layers each one on top of the last, the stomach wall gradually enfolds the food. Part of the stomach's function, after all, is to bring the food into contact with the stomach wall, in which the glands that produce gastric juice for digestion are located. Real and continued contact is facilitated by strong muscular waves in the stomach wall that create kneading movements. The moment food touches the stomach wall, the kneading begins, brought about partly through reflex action but mostly through the effect of the hormone gastrin in the bloodstream.

Gastrin stimulates both the secretion of gastric juice and the muscular waves (tonic contractions). The muscular waves cause the stomach contents to become thoroughly mixed and bathed in gastric juice; they begin at the top of the stomach (the fundus) and travel the length of the entire organ in a progressive contraction called peristalsis that ceases only at the pyloric sphincter, the entry to the duodenum. The antrum and the pylorus in fact together constitute the major method of kneading the food, the antrum forcing the food towards the pylorus, the pylorus restricting the exit of the food and so squeezing it. This is the most important area of the stomach's function, in relation to which the fundus and the corpus of the stomach may be seen as simply a reservoir for food awaiting processing by the antrum and pylorus.

How quickly the stomach empties depends on the kind of food that is eaten, the combination of foods, how the acid-base balance is affected and, most of all, on the overall quantity of food consumed.

Fat inhibits gastric motility.　The presence of fat in the duodenum immediately causes the muscular contractions of the stomach wall to slow and weaken. The mechanism by which this is achieved depends on the secretion of enterogastrone, a hormone (actually, a complex of hormones) that is released into the bloodstream and travels back up to the stomach to inhibit both the secretion of gastric juice and gastric motility.

Once gastric motility is reduced, food automatically clings to the stomach wall for a longer time, and the enzymatic reaction has a longer period in which to occur – as is most advantageous for the digestion of protein. High-protein foods contain large proportions of fats; foods low in protein contain little or no fats. This is a measure of the natural relationship between protein and fat.

Cereals do not contain much in the way of fat (1.7–7.1 per cent by volume) in spite of their relatively high protein content (7.4–12.6 per cent). This is why it is a good idea to combine cereals with fat: the protein is much easier to digest. Vegetables, which are difficult to digest because of their solid structure, also greatly benefit from the addition of fat in the form of salad dressing or mayonnaise.

The Passage of Food Through the Stomach

Filling the stomach.　There are many misconceptions about how the stomach deals with the food that is eaten. Most people seem to imagine the stomach as some kind of cauldron in which food simmers within a seething stock of gastric juice. But the stomach is a highly mobile organ, and digestion relies on its inner surface only. Food in the stomach gravitates downwards under its own weight, to accumulate in the antrum. There, through peristalsis the stomach wall squeezes it against itself and the entrance to the duodenum.

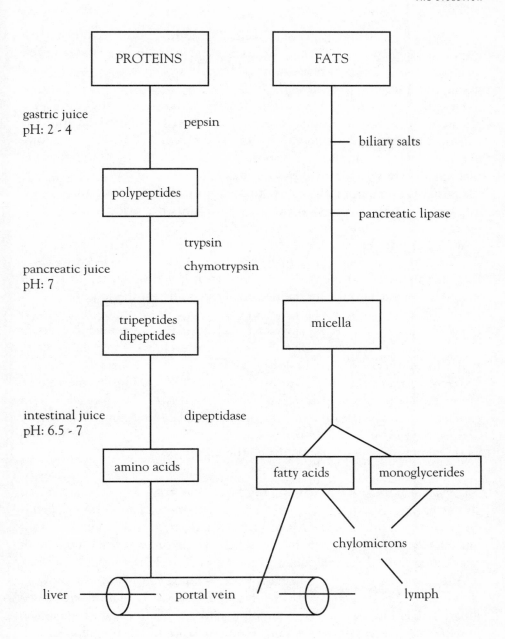

A schematic diagram of the digestion and reabsorption of proteins and fats.

The stomach gradually fills from the outside inwards, layer by layer, according to the sequence of the meal. What is eaten first clings to the stomach wall; whatever is eaten next lies on top of it; and what is eaten last is located in the middle of the stomach.

How the stomach is gradually filled has been the subject of considerable research with x-rays and using laboratory animals. The animal experiments consisted of feeding the individuals successively with coloured foods, allowing digestion to get under way, putting the animals to sleep, and freezing them before autopsy. The results were clear.

Peristalsis in the stomach ensures that the pulpy chyme is well mixed with gastric juice. Digested food is pressed on towards the pylorus and out, in order to make room for food not yet digested.

We shall now consider a traditional four-course lunch consisting of a starter, a soup or side-dish, a main course, and a dessert. The starter will form the first layer in the stomach, the side-dish will lie on top of it, then the main course, and finally the dessert. Depending on the kind of food, a lot of time may be required for each of these contents separately to mix with the gastric juice – and, as we have seen, such a mixing is essential in order to kill inimical bacteria, to stabilize the sugars, and to break down the protein. If the mixing takes place too slowly (as is all too often the case), there is a risk of fermentation inside the stomach (or less commonly thereafter). Fermentation in this way is possible only in areas of the stomach not in contact with the gastric juice, notably in the middle of the stomach. A sugary dessert or fruit on a full stomach always causes fermentation because the sugar cannot make contact with the gastric juice.

The empty stomach.   A very commonly asked question is: Does the stomach always have to be empty before we start a new meal? The answer depends on what the stomach had in it to begin with. The stomach empties itself only slowly: after heavy, fatty meals, it can take six or even seven hours, but after eating easily digestible food it may take a much shorter time.

After a night's rest, the stomach is always empty. If it is not, we know all about it: we feel nauseous, our breath is foul, and we have a thickly coated tongue. An empty stomach is very receptive to the next food: the food enters in sequence and empties in the same sequence without any problem. Even if there is some residual food left in the stomach, there should be no problem if the residue allows itself to be combined with the new meal. But when this is not the case – as when a high-protein meal that has not been fully digested is joined by a meal rich in starch or sugar – a bad combination of foods is formed in the stomach . . . and the fireworks start.

a

b

1. starter
2. soup or side-dish
3. main course
4. dessert
5. air bubble

1. *The starter has left the stomach.*
2. *The remains of the soup or side-dish reach the final area of the stomach.*
3. *The main course arrives at the antrum.*
4. *The dessert accumulates progressively in the middle of the stomach, not touching the stomach wall despite the peristalsis in the fundus and the corpus: there is a danger of fermentation.*

c

d

The food leaves the stomach in the same sequence in which it first arrived there.

A stomach that is too full. One of the most frequent causes of digestive problems involving internal fermentation and toxic degradation is undoubtedly the consumption of too much food at one time, whether the food is all of one type or a ripe old mixture. The stomach is not actually all that large, and we should try to accustom ourselves to the idea that a moderate amount of food should be enough for any meal. 'Little but often' is a well-known description of good eating habits – and it is quite right, and should be

This illustration shows a stomach in which there is still food left from a previous meal (4), even as new food is being ingested (1, 2, 3). As far as the stomach is concerned, there is no difference between the last layer of the previous meal and the first layer of the new meal. If they are compatible, there should be no risk of digestive problems. Foods that can be combined may be eaten one after another without the stomach's having to be empty in between. Foods that should not be combined, such as high-protein and high-starch foods, should always be eaten on an empty stomach in order to ensure separation from each other.

brought firmly to mind whenever stomach and digestive complaints occur. It really is a pity that most people wilfully ignore this rule and insist on having three or even two meals at set times per day. Actually by eating so few times a day, we are encouraging ourselves to eat too much on each occasion. It is logical, of course, in that we need a certain quantity of food every day, but for the stomach there is a considerable difference between whether that same quantity is spread over two meals or five.

Several biologists have pointed out that an ideal volume for a meal that could be digested smoothly might be somewhere in the region of ¼ litre (about ½ pint); this represents a quantity that does not cause the exterior wall of the stomach to expand. Double that quantity, and the stomach wall does expand, but still within acceptable margins. Six times the initial quantity (1.5 litres), however, is just about the maximum a stomach can take at full expansion, and we may assume the stomach suffers from it. The elasticity of the stomach wall is reduced, perhaps permanently, and the abdomen ('belly') begins to sag.

A volume of 1.5 litres (about 3 pints) is very difficult for the stomach to cope with. The risk of fermentation in the middle of the stomach is high: there is just too much material for it all to be mixed well with the gastric juice. Eating food that is rich in water, however, greatly reduces the volume once it reaches the stomach because water leaves the stomach faster – this is why the maintenance of the acid-base balance is so important to the diet.

Ideally, any one meal should not exceed 500–600 grams (1–1½ pounds) in overall weight.

The shape of the stomach.   If one eats too much food in one go, and does not take any account of food combining, the stomach becomes heavily laden and begins to bulge. There are three common shapes into which the stomach distends: in this book they are described as the hooked stomach, the long stomach, and the moose-horn stomach.

The hooked stomach occurs quite frequently, although it is perhaps the least similar to the original stomach shape. Much of the outer wall is vertical so that about half of the stomach is almost cylindrical, before curving into a rather badly kinked hook.

The long stomach is found more in women than in men. The stomach streches downwards a surprising distance, to the fourth lumbar vertebra or even lower. The food accumulates in a lump at the bottom (as it does in the hooked stomach), and the fundus and corpus are then all too suitable locations for fermentation to occur.

The moose-horn stomach is caused by the distended coils of the small intestine as the quantity of food passes through them, pressing up against the stomach from beneath.

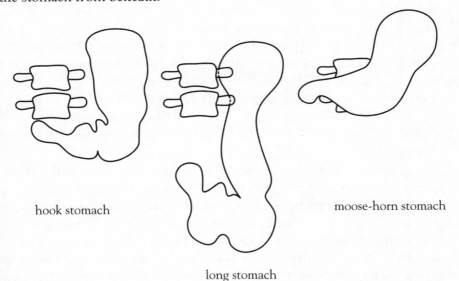

hook stomach

long stomach

moose-horn stomach

Distended stomach shapes.

Drinking during meals.   Drinking during meals has little or no effect on the digestion of solid food for the simple reason that liquids are filtered off much faster. When we eat soup, the water of the soup flows straight down special folds in the shorter curved inner wall of the stomach, and on to the pylorus: liquids always take the most direct path consistent with gravity. Once the liquid has quickly drained away, the rest of the food is left in the form of a usefully pliable mass.

Drinking does not dilute the gastric juice (as is sometimes suggested). From the stomach wall, gastric juice is produced whenever necessary and in whatever quantity is necessary. Indeed, people who have a peptic ulcer suffer from overproduction of gastric juice. Wouldn't it be just a little too easy if they could cure all their problems just by drinking a glass of water to dilute the gastric juice in their stomachs! The nutritional biologists J. F. de Wijn and W. T. J. M. Hekkens have no truck with any such notions: 'It is a figment of the imagination to suppose that drinking during a meal might be harmful because it causes the gastric juice to be diluted.'

During meals that consist largely of cereals or bread, however, it is not advisable to take a drink while there is still food in the mouth, for drinking makes chewing impossible. For similar reasons, dunking bits of bread in tea, coffee, or any other liquid is not to be recommended: the bread becomes so soft that it cannot be properly chewed, and the possibility of predigestion in the mouth is lost.

There is one golden rule in relation to drinking: drink when thirsty. But what kind of drink we take may also affect the digestion. We can always drink still (non-carbonated) spring water, which has no effect at all on digestion. Soft drinks, cola, beer and wine are altogether different. Cola has a very high degree of acidity (pH 1.9) and disrupts the digestion of starch by making the saliva more acid. It also interferes with the digestion of high-protein foods by inhibiting the gastric juice (acid inhibits acid).

Real health fanatics eat their soup at the end of the meal (which does not make much sense) or tend to drink only before or long after they have eaten.

Air in the stomach.   It is all too easy for an air bubble to form in the uppermost part of the stomach, the fundus. Bubbles are caused by swallowing air while eating, and especially while eating too rapidly. Both of these factors explain why babies have to be burped. A person who eats too much too fast creates a large air bubble in the stomach. As the stomach takes on its muscular peristalsis to knead the food, and while the pylorus is still closed, an unpleasantly tense sensation is felt. If the lower oesophageal segment allows the air to escape upwards, the person belches. Nervous tension can increase this process. Acid indigestion is what happens when gastric juice is also brought up out of the stomach and into the lower portion of the oesophagus. Fermentation or toxic degradation in the stomach can make the situation even worse as gases accumulate and pressurize within the stomach.

Emptying the stomach. The stomach is a kind of storage depot in which food is stowed until a fair proportion of the protein has been digested. It is also the location at which the food is brought to the correct temperature. Food that is too hot is cooled, and food that is too cold is warmed, to body temperature. The enzymatic processes of digestion take place only at the correct temperature.

How long the stomach takes to empty depends on a number of factors, of which the most decisive is the total quantity of food eaten. In addition, there is the type of food, the composition of the menu (including whether an attempt at harmonious food combining has been made), the state of the body's acid-base balance, how well the food is eaten (and especially chewed), the current state of the digestive system, and so forth. If the meal consists largely of fruit, digestion will be quite rapid. Adding whipped cream to the fruit, however, slows digestion down. Raw vegetables and boiled food both take a longer digestion time. And high-protein foods (such as meat and fish dishes, dishes including leguminous vegetables, and dishes prepared with soy products) demand a great deal of time for digestion.

A stomach containing around 900 millilitres (2 pints) of food belonging to a traditional-style menu takes between six and seven hours to digest. Particularly heavy, fatty foods may stay in the stomach for much longer, and may therefore be subject to the risk of fermentation and toxic degradation.

The Duodenum

The duodenum may be described as the centre of digestion. This is where the main digestion of protein, starch and fat takes place. In relation to what happens here, the disgestion of some starch in the mouth and the digestion of a proportion of protein in the stomach may both be considered no more than contributing to a process of predigestion. Similarly, the later and much more limited digestive processes in the small and large intestines may be described as post-digestion. What all this means is that the overall digestive process is highly complex.

One other remarkable process occurs in the duodenum and has consider-able relevance to food combining. The food contents received from the stomach bathed in acids are brought to acid-alkali neutrality. Pancreatic juice ducted into the duodenum contains water and sodium bicarbonate, a substance that has a considerable capacity for combining with acids. The environment of the stomach is strongly acidic, but that in the duodenum and intestines (under the influence of pancreatic juice and intestinal juice) is alkaline or only very slightly acidic (pH 6.5–8), as it is required to be if the local enzymes are to function properly. The pylorus does not open to allow food to leave the stomach and enter the duodenum until the correct pH value has been attained in the duodenum.

The neutralizing process actually begins at the very end of the stomach, and takes place over a total linear distance of only about 10 centimetres (4 inches). But the pylorus emits only a very small amount of food into the duodenum at a time, which is one reason why the stomach empties so slowly. This is, if anything, an advantage, however, for it allows digestion to take place in the duodenum at a comparative slow and therefore thorough pace.

Every food contains protein, carbohydrates and fat. Even if a person eats only one type of food, these three constituents are always present. But the pancreas cannot secrete three different enzymes simultaneously, one to cope with each, because there is only one duct linking the pancreas to the duodenum. So the pancreas effectively chooses the order in which the food constituents are to be digested, depending on the proportions of those constituents in the food. Following a high-protein meal, the enzyme protease is produced and secreted first; following a meal rich in starch, it is the enzyme amylase that comes first; and following a meal rich in fats it is pancreatic lipase.

The function of the pancreas in secreting its enzymes may be disrupted by inappropriate combinations of foods. Disruption may occur, for instance, if several different foods are consumed at once, and in the form of chyme enter the duodenum in unusually mixed composition (containing, perhaps, as much protein as starch, or – worse – some protein or starch that has been hardly touched by earlier digestive processes).

Bile entering the duodenum from the gall bladder does not contain any digestive enzymes but serves as an emulsifier. The structure of the fat in the food is altered so that pancreatic lipase triglyceride splits up to form monoglyceride and free fatty acids.

It is the hormone cholecystokinin that stimulates the gall bladder to secrete bile; pancreozymine stimulates enzyme secretion in the pancreas. Bile is also secreted in some quantity by the liver, and flows with bile from the gall bladder to the duodenum. The presence of fats and peptides in the stomach and duodenum thus effectively causes bile to be produced and

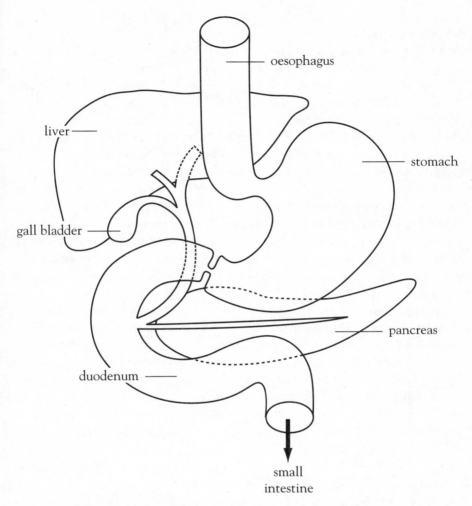

oesophagus

liver

stomach

gall bladder

pancreas

duodenum

small
intestine

A schematic diagram showing the relationship of the duodenum to the pancreas, stomach, liver, and gall bladder.

secreted, as does eating egg yolk, because it stimulates a strong contraction of the gall bladder.

The Small Intestine

The small intestine has two sections which merge into each other almost imperceptibly. The first part is the jejunum, the second the ileum. To all intents and purposes, digestion is completed in the small intestine (and the process there may therefore be described as post-digestion). The nutrients and the other constituents such as minerals and vitamins into which the food has been broken down during digestion are now taken through the intestinal wall and absorbed or transported in the bloodstream.

Let us now briefly review digestion as it has been presented so far, noting in particular a number of significant physiological aspects.

Starch undergoes predigestion in the mouth through the agency of the salivary enzyme ptyalin. In the stomach, the sugars already released are stabilized by gastric juice to prevent fermentation. No further digestion of starch takes place in the stomach. In the duodenum, however, the complex sugars that constitute starch undergo further breakdown by pancreatic amylase to become disaccharides. And these disaccharides receive the final digestive treatment in the small intestine, for in the mucous membranes of the intestinal wall are glands that produce various enzymes: maltase, which breaks maltose down to glucose; saccharase, which breaks saccharose (cane or beet sugar) down to fructose; and lactase, which breaks lactose (milk sugar) down to galactose.

The digestion of protein begins in the stomach, where the hydrochloric acid secreted there activates pepsinogens to form all or most of eight different pepsins. This is the first stage of protein breakdown. In the duodenum, pancreatic juice converts trypsinogen and chymotrypsinogen to trypsin and chymotrypsin, and these enzymes then break down the protein into di-peptides. It is in the small intestine that the peptides are finally broken down into individual amino acids under the influence of the enzyme dipeptidase. Various resorption systems then transport the amino acids from within the intestine to the bloodstream.

Fat is always the last to undergo digestion. Babies predigest some milk fat in the stomach, but for adults fat digestion takes place virtually solely in the duodenum, as effected by bile and pancreatic lipase. In the small intestine, fatty acids and monoglycerides are absorbed by the mucous membrane of the jejunum, and biliary salts are absorbed only in the ileum.

The small intestine is known for its forceful peristaltic waves which not only press the food on its continuous path but bring it into good contact with the intestinal wall, thereby accomplishing the various processes of digestion described.

The Large Intestine

The large intestine consists of the caecum, from which the appendix dangles, the ascending colon, the transverse colon, the descending colon, and the rectum, which ends at the anus.

It has various functions, specifically the resorption of water and mineral salts, the compaction and excretion of faeces, the synthesis of certain vitamins (notably vitamin B_{12}), and the final sorting out of digestive difficulties. The human organism works extremely efficiently; nothing need be wasted. Even as water and salts are undergoing reabsorption from the large intestine, a final endeavour to digest nutrients not already digested is in progress.

Much of what the large intestine does concerns controlled fermentation, in which the caecum plays a prominent part. The small intestine injects small quantities of chyme into the caecum via the ileo-caecal valve. There, in the initial 'chamber' of the large intestine, a fermentation process takes place under the influence of the bacillus *Escherichia coli*; this is where the intestinal flora chiefly reside.

The natural process of fermentation – as found for instance in the large intestine of anthropoid apes – is rarely found in humans, at least in advanced countries, because of the persistent consumption of the wrong foods. In most people, the large intestine has instead degenerated into a receptacle for wastes and the results of fermentation and toxic degradation from earlier in the sequence of digestion. The consequent effects are constipation, intestinal diseases and disorders, the distension of the intestinal walls through gas and stretching, and a great deal of discomfort.

One of the great goals of food combining is to improve the working of the large intestine, an organ in which, as Dr Nolfi rightly says, 'death lurks'.

My years of experience in food combining, together with my knowledge of the effects of enemas, fasting, and various other practices that have to do with diet and digestion, have proved to my own satisfaction that problem-free digestion is the fundamental basis of good health. In fact, the better the digestive function, the less is the actual need for food. Those who have broken through this vicious circle are able to derive a great deal of energy from only a small quantity of food. And the use of a smaller quantity of food in turn means less waste, less poisoning, less 'acidity', less energy used in dealing with food, and the relief and pleasure of smooth digestion and good overall health.

Intestinal Gases

Gas and wind in the intestines is produced by fermentation and by degradation of food matter (whether toxic residues make an additional appearance or not). Eating food in quantities that are excessive or that is too concentrated to maintain a proper acid-base balance, and eating it without attention to harmonious food combining, causes digestive problems. The complex digestive system, with its many enzymatic and hormonal processes, is simply unable to digest the food in an optimal fashion. Undigested residues are left behind – mostly starch, sugar, and protein residues. Starch and sugar start to ferment, but protein residues begin degradation.

There are a number of different processes of fermentation, mostly named after the result of the process (like alcoholic, lactic, butyric, acetic, propionic, and so forth). The intestine forms a perfect site for fermentation processes: the temperature is ideal, the appropriate bacteria are present, and there is a comparatively alkaline environment (a high pH value).

In natural circumstances, fermentation should indeed take place in the large intestine – but in the caecum, after which any food residue that remains in the chyme can be digested in due course and in its proper place. This important process is most often disrupted by fermentation and degradation at an earlier stage, causing very unpleasant effects.

Residues of protein stimulate the growth of certain bacteria, unbalancing the equilibrium of the intestinal flora but also converting the residues into gases, some of which can be extremely poisonous. In addition to nitrogen and oxygen, they may contain hydrogen and methane, although the overall smell is mostly determined by the proportional presence of amines and hydrogen sulphide. Some of the intestinal gases may be taken up by the bloodstream and eventually exhaled through the lungs as bad breath.

The bacteria do not convert food residues only into gases, however, but can also produce toxic substances. Fourteen potentially serious toxins have been detected in human intestines and faeces.

In addition to flatulence, gases in the intestines may cause a condition of inflation by which the contents of the abdomen (the 'belly') distend outwards and upwards, pushing against the stomach so that the diaphragm is put under pressure. This pressure may then be relayed by the diaphragm to the heart and lungs. In this way, intestinal gas may be responsible for heart palpitations and shortness of breath.

When no pathological cause can be found, intestinal gases are caused by bad digestion. In the stomach they are produced mainly by the fermentation of sugars in the middle of the organ or by disruption to the breakdown of protein. Pressure via the diaphragm on the heart and lungs is even stronger when caused by gas in the stomach than it is when caused by intestinal gas.

Latent fermentation and degradation processes can cause acute symptoms after a meal. This is because a full stomach transmits impulses to the intestines increasing peristalsis there, causing a very heavy sensation in the abdomen and, in some people, a sudden urge to defecate.

Allergic Reaction

People who know they suffer from a food allergy may well experience a rapid improvement in the condition if they concentrate on food combining.

This may sound presumptuous, not to say unbelievable, in that allergy is a disorder of the immune system and has no direct relationship with digestion. But with food combining, it is not the cause of the allergy that is removed but the factors that induce the reaction. Eating different foods at random and all mixed up creates a disrupted digestion: gases and toxins are formed, and protein residues remain in the intestines. These are absorbed through the intestinal wall into the bloodstream, causing an allergic reaction.

Masked allergies (allergies of which the major allergen is difficult to pinpoint or unknown) are relatively easy to cure by food combining. An allergy test may show that a person is not allergic to bread, meat, or cheese, but suffers an allergic reaction when eating bread with meat or cheese. This is an allergy not to the foods themselves but to the poisonous substances or protein residues that enter the bloodstream because of the combination of foods.

Harmonious food combining results in perfect digestion. Perfect digestion improves the metabolism as a whole, making allergic reactions generally less likely.

CHAPTER 4

FOOD COMBINING:
GOOD AND BAD COMBINATIONS

One of the most common causes of poor digestion, prevalent all over the country, is the consumption of combinations of foods that are incompatible. The fact that just about everybody chooses to forget the limited capabilities of the digestive enzymes and eats pretty well anything at any time is responsible in large measure for the indigestion from which nearly everyone suffers more or less continually. Evidence for this is that good food combining stops indigestion altogether. Nonetheless, good food combining only improves digestion – it does not end it – if the indigestion is partly caused by other factors. If worry is a major factor, for example, the worry has to disappear before digestion can return to normal. And we should be aware that worry together with bad combinations of foods causes worse indigestion than worry together with harmonious combinations of foods.

Adapted from Dr Herbert M. Shelton: Food Combining . . . Made Easy,
San Antonio, Texas, 1951.

As we know, the five nutrients in food are protein, fat, sugar, starch, and acids, and all are directly involved in food combining. Other substances – roughage (dietary fibre), vitamins, minerals, water, aromatic substances, and so on – may also be conducive to good digestion. The body's acid-base balance may, for example, feel the benefit of consuming metallic elements and water. But these substances have no influence over the effect of the combination of foods, good or bad.

Some nutrients in combination react against each other, either preventing one or other from imparting its full benefit or disrupting the smooth function of the digestive process generally. Foods that contain large proportions of such incompatible nutrients should not be eaten in combination at all: these are not appropriate to food combining. Nutrients that go together well, on the other hand, are what food combining is all about.

By now we should all be familiar with the pentagon that shows the good and the bad combinations of food types (see p. 13). There are six bad combinations and four good combinations on the pentagon. In practice, however, there are more. (Mathematically, the five nutrients can be combined in pairs in more than 3,100 different ways.) Here, I will stick to the original ten, plus one or two others that can be mentioned separately.

Opponents of food combining may point out that every type of food tends to have at least four nutrients in it, and not uncommonly five. They usually state quite firmly that all these nutrients are digested simultaneously. They are right, up to a point. Every type of food does contain protein, fat and acid, and usually contains either starch or sugar but may contain both. So even if we eat only one type of food, without variation, the digestive system does have four or five nutrients to contend with. But not at the same time. They are digested in a specific sequence.

It has already been pointed out that the nutrients occur in certain proportions in foods, and that there is nearly always a dominant nutrient. The proportions of nutrients are thus of great significance, central to the overall composition of every food. In food combining, the objective should be to retain those proportions. So, for instance, it is not the fact that protein and starch may be combined in a meal that is important so much as the ratio of protein to starch in it.

In many foods, such as potatoes, protein and starch are both present. The ratio of one to the other is so favourable that digestion is not interfered with. But if we were to eat meat with the potatoes, the overall proportions would be completely different, and so unfavourable in their effects that the combination can be described as bad.

Foods that are evolutionarily suited to human digestion always have favourable proportions of nutrients. So in many agricultural products – cereals, milk products, leguminous vegetables and soya, for example – the protein-starch ratio is unfavourable. And in industrial products – such as sausages, biscuits, soft drinks, puddings, chocolate and processed meats – the ratio is pretty well arbitrary or random. Eating only one kind of food, without variation, ensures excellent digestion. Whenever combining foods, it is necessary to take their composition into account in order to be aware of the proportions of nutrients in them. To eat a random selection of different foods is to confront the digestive process with several dominant nutrients: digestion becomes difficult, and occasionally even impossible.

As an example of a popular lunchtime dish, let us look at chicken with rice.

In graph A, protein is dominant, and supported by fat: protein-fat is a natural combination. In graph B, starch is dominant. In graph C, protein and starch vie for dominance.

By combining foods we change the proportions of the nutrients they contain – proportions that are central to food combining. Knowing what the proportions are, it is possible to put together meals that are good combinations of foods. Many combinations hardly change the porportions at all, allowing digestion to take place smoothly and efficiently perhaps in spite of the fact that several different foods may be eaten together.

Combining different foods can result in good, problematical, and truly bad combinations. Dr Shelton chose to distinguish a fourth category: excellent combinations. I have felt obliged to reject that notion because no combination of food types can improve on a diet that consists of one food only, without variation.

Food combining corresponds to dietary rules that are applied to allow us to eat several different foods in one meal, or even one dish, with unimpaired digestion.

The health and condition of the digestive system also has an important role to play in the success or otherwise of food combining. People who for one reason or another have weak digestive systems cannot help but suffer digestive problems whenever they eat several types of food at the same time. Good combinations of foods cause only minor problems, but difficult or truly bad combinations may have serious consequences.

Such people should benefit from a diet of rather staid dishes or, better still, from a diet of the same food all the time. People whose digestive systems are strong experience few problems, even when they are not particularly careful about what they eat in combination. They can tolerate many of the combinations that are labelled difficult or problematical, in which the good proportions of nutrients are exceeded but only by a slight margin. Difficult or problematical combinations, then, may still be digested reasonably well by those with strong enough digestive systems.

Bad combinations are bad because the proportions of nutrients in them make them unsuitable for anybody to eat. People whose digestive systems are particularly strong and vigorous may be able to tolerate them for some time, but only at the expense of considerable energy in digesting.

It has already been pointed out that food combining is not an end in itself but is one of several elements of a healthy dietary regime. It is possible to eat a good combination of foods and yet disrupt the body's acid-base balance.

Meat with vegetables is a good combination, but a lot of meat eaten with only few vegetables distorts the acid-base balance. Digestion becomes more difficult, and too many acids are formed during metabolism.

Something else that can spoil digestion even with a good combination of foods is overeating: eat too much food, and no matter whether it is all of the same type, digestion suffers.

In relation to food combining, then, it is useful also to take into account the acid-base balance, to restrict the amount of food eaten in any one meal, to eat as slowly as possible (especially when eating fruit), to concentrate on what is being eaten but at the same time to avoid thinking too much during a meal, and above all to enjoy the food in the excellent combination in which it has been prepared. If all these parameters are observed, food combining will turn out to be the blessing it ought to be.

This chapter is devoted hereafter to bad, good and problematical combinations of food, in that order.

BAD COMBINATIONS

Combining Protein and Starch

The combination of protein and starch is one of the most common bad ones. Particularly well-attested forms are bread and cheese, meat and potatoes, chicken and rice, peanut-butter (or other nut-based spread) sandwiches, and so on. Meat and meat products, fish, cheese, bread, cereals and potatoes are the mainstays of industrialized foods. They have an ancient tradition as such, and represent the heart of the modern food economy.

It may be said that most of these foods are not suitable for human consumption – but it is not realistic to think that we can do without them. Many nutritionists have pressed for a reduction in animal protein in order to cut down on the consumption of meat. But a shift in ideas is becoming apparent at the moment. Low-protein foods have taken on a new popularity, resulting in increased interest in fruit and vegetables. Yet for those who stick to the traditional diet of meat, fish, cheese, bread, and so forth, there is a considerable advantage in watching out for the better combinations of foods.

Everyone knows how a hearty traditional meal can lie heavy on the stomach afterwards, but only few people are aware that this heaviness derives from bad food combining, and that it can easily be prevented by not eating high-protein food and starch-rich food at the same time.

The protein-starch combination was particularly favoured by the old school of nutritionists (including Doctors Hay and Shelton, and others). Indeed, Dr Hay based his entire theory upon this very combination, wrong as it is, and it was later adopted also by Dr Shelton. Why they should have done so, and so misguidedly, demands an explanation.

The old theory had it that starch is digested in the mouth by the salivary enzyme ptyalin, an enzyme that required an alkaline environment in order to function. That is not the case: ptyalin actually requires a mildly acidic environment. But because protein is digested in the stomach by the enzyme pepsin in a highly acidic environment, it was thought that the digestion of starch was impossible there, and starch was therefore only digested in the mouth. This is also untrue: the digestion of starch in the mouth is indeed halted by gastric juice once the starch arrives in the stomach, but resumes again when the starch reaches the duodenum.

It was also thought that starch in the stomach begins to ferment because the alkaline-requiring ptyalin was destroyed. But fermentation cannot actually occur in an acidic environment. The gastric acids do not cause the released sugars to ferment, as Hay and Shelton thought. On the contrary, the gastric juice stabilizes the sugars so they cannot ferment – completely the opposite effect. No doubt some will now say that a bloated feeling in the stomach is quite common. It certainly is – but the feeling is not caused by the juxtaposition of sugars and gastric juice, as the old school imagined.

As we know, the stomach is filled layer by layer from the outside in. If we overeat, part of the food remains in the middle of the upper area of the stomach for too long, not coming into contact with the inner stomach wall, and so not being mixed with gastric juice. When this happens, the sugars start to ferment, and gas accumulates.

It is totally understandable that the theory of food combining used never to be accepted by classical dieticians: the principle, as stated by its proponents in those days, was incorrect. Food combining, as outlined in this book, however, conforms in every detail with modern physiological science.

No foods have a pH value of 7 or higher – neutral and alkaline foods do not exist. If they did, they wouldn't last long. All foods contain acids, and it is the acids that destroy bacteria, so ensuring that the food keeps for as long as possible. The storage life of food thus depends totally on the acid content. (The acids described here are free acids, and not the bound or conjugate acids that determine the acid-base balance.)

When we eat starchy food, predigestion takes place in the mouth. As we chew, the starch is partly converted first into disaccharides and, if we chew on long enough, into monosaccharides. If all we eat is starchy foods, the sugar that is released is stabilized by the gastric juice in the stomach. All foods contain protein, if sometimes only in a tiny quantity. This protein is partly digested in the stomach.

The secretion of gastric juice depends upon a number of factors. At a maximum, secretion of hydrochloric acid gives the gastric juice a pH value of around 1, which is extremely acidic. The type of food that is being digested modifies this acidity to a pH value of anything between 2 and 4 as a buffer effect: pepsins function at their best at this degree of acidity.

According to the proponents of the old school, gastric juice becomes neutral if starchy foods such as potatoes or bread are eaten, in which case ptyalin can then continue its digestive activity on starch. But this is all wrong. If we were to eat only cauliflower or courgettes, mildly acidic vegetables with a pH value of about 5.9, the pH value of the gastric acid would remain at around 4, and the available protein would still be broken down.

Let us look at bread and cheese, firstly at how they are digested separately, and secondly at how they are digested when eaten together. We shall be able to understand then why they should never be eaten together.

When we eat bread, or bread and butter, the starch is partly broken down to sugars in the mouth by the saliva. When the food reaches the stomach, the gastric juice secreted is of a type that is geared to cope with such starch-rich material. The protein in the bread (about 7 per cent) is partly broken down by pepsins in the acidic environment. Those sugars that have already been released during chewing are stabilized in the stomach, so preventing them from fermenting. Gradually, the stomach contents are passed on to the duodenum where the starch, protein and fat are digested one after the other.

When we eat cheese by itself, the well-chewed cheese proceeds to the stomach, where the gastric juice secreted is of a type that is geared to cope with high-protein food (around 25–35 per cent protein), remaining quite acidic.

So what happens when we eat bread with cheese? The digestive process is pretty much the same as with bread alone: the digestion of starch and protein happens virtually simultaneously and, as we have seen, can do so without difficulty because there are effectively two separate digestive processes, one in the mouth and the other in the stomach. All the same, experience tells us that the combination is not a good one.

By eating bread with cheese, we are putting together two dominant nutrients: starch and protein. Because neither bread nor cheese can satisfy the stomach, it is all too easy to eat too much of both of them. But too much of these foods in the stomach makes for fermentation, because of the excess starch. The presence of two dominant nutrients in the stomach causes digestion to become difficult: the process takes place slowly and in-completely. The quantity also adds to the difficulty.

Thereafter, digestion becomes even more problematical as the material proceeds to the duodenum, the small intestine and the large intestine. The pancreas in particular has a difficult task, for large quantities of protein, starch and fat are present all at the same time. Digestion is necessarily incomplete. Part of the protein begins to degrade; part of the starch begins to ferment. The intestine provides an environment suited to fermentation, and the process continues apace in virtually ideal conditions. The result is an intestine bloated with gases, a situation that is specifically caused by the bad combination of protein and starch.

High-protein foods and starchy foods should not be combined. The protein-starch combination distorts the acid-base balance and makes diges-tion difficult. If two types of protein are involved, digestion becomes even more problematical.

Examples of protein-starch combinations include:

bread and cheese
meat and potatoes
chicken and rice
cheese and spaghetti
meatballs and chips/French fries
fish and potato croquettes

Combining Starch and Sugar

The combination of starch and sugar is almost as common as that of protein and starch. Fillings in sandwiches are generally sweet, except when sliced meat or cheese is used instead. Sweet tastes are extremely popular: sugar consumption in Europe varies between 35 and 55 kilograms (75–120 pounds) per person per year. Bread with jam, jelly, chocolate, sweet spread, syrup, honey, bananas, and so on, causes fermentation. Pastry is always a combination of starch, sugar and fat. Honey-cakes, raisin bread, custard tarts, doughnuts, and other such delicacies are all upsetting to the digestion.

These much-loved sweet foods are the direct cause of the obesity evident in a large proportion of the populations of advanced countries. Weak abdominal muscles are often said to be responsible for a paunch, but this is to ignore the fact that the weakness of the muscles is not so much the cause as the result. A 'beer belly' is caused by the fermentation of sugars and not by the quantity of liquid consumed.

But how can starch and sugar represent such a bad combination if one of the main effects of gastric juice is to stabilize sugars, so preventing fermentation? The answer is in the relative proportions of the nutrients. To combine starch and sugar is to juxtapose two dominant nutrients that are digested in totally different ways: we are mixing two different digestion processes.

When we eat a food rich in sugar (like a spoonful of honey, a ripe banana, or a lump of sugar), digestion takes place quite fast: the breaking down of disaccharides to become monosaccharides happens smoothly and effort-lessly. In the stomach the sugar is stabilized by the gastric juice, proceeding intact to the duodenum and onward, so that absorption can occur in the small intestine.

But we have already seen how the digestion of a food rich in starch takes place slowly, mainly because of the presence also of protein and fat. If we eat starch and sugar in one meal, or even one dish, we run the risk that part of the sugar will end up in the fermentation zone of the stomach, in the middle, away from the gastric juice, and will begin to ferment. Slow and incomplete digestion lead to the presence of undigested disaccharides and starch residues in the chyme within the intestines, where further fermentation takes place, inevitably resulting in intestinal bloating.

Imagine a jam sandwich passing through the digestive process. If it is by itself, things may not be too difficult. But if there is more than one sandwich, there is the risk of fermentation. The retarded stomach function is confronted with too large a quantity of sugar to be mixed with gastric juice for the sugars to be stabilized.

As we know, fruit, a sweet dessert, or any other type of sweet food should not be eaten on a full stomach. Whatever is last to be eaten settles itself in the middle of the stomach, far from the stomach wall, in the fermentation zone.

Examples of starch-sugar combinations include:

a sandwich with a sweet filling
bread with a banana or other high-sugar fruit
bread and honey
a pie or tart with a sweet filling
raisin bread
a honey-cake
waffles
cakes
pastries

Combining Starch and Acid

The predigestion of starch occurs in the mouth as a result of the presence of the salivary enzyme ptyalin, which works in an environment that is mildly acidic (pH 5.5–7). If we eat food with a degree of acidity higher than 5.5, the saliva becomes too acid and the ptyalin has no effect. Exactly the same thing happens if we drink acidic beverages with a meal, for they too are mixed with saliva in the mouth.

If the starch is not predigested, digestion has to start in the duodenum, under the auspices of the pancreas. It is a heavy burden for the pancreas, and there remains a risk that part of the starch will not be broken down and that sugar residues will undergo fermentation in the intestine, causing intestinal bloating and flatulence. It is always in our own interests to try to make sure that starch is properly predigested – and people with weak digestive systems in particular should address themselves to this need.

It is all too easy to eat starch and acid together, for very few people know enough to be aware that the combination eliminates predigestion and may cause digestive problems. Sourdough bread, for example, much lauded around the world, is a starch-acid combination. The sourdough in fact makes the saliva so acid as to render the predigestion of starch impossible. In consequence, sourdough bread is itself difficult to digest. Worse, if we eat sourdough bread with honey or jam, we are presenting our digestive system with a starch-acid-sugar combination; if we eat it instead with cheese, cold meat or nut spread, it is a starch-acid-protein combination. Eating organic food is frequently contrary to the principles of food combining.

Bread together with fruit is similarly a bad combination in general, for fruit always contains acids and renders the saliva acid too. Certainly, some fruits are more acidic than others, and the more acidic a fruit is, the more difficult it is to combine with starch. But even sweet fruit can have a high degree of acidity (like bananas, with a pH value of 3.8).

The combination of bread or potatoes with acidic fruit and vegetables like tomatoes or rhubarb should also be avoided. Combinations of starchy foods with vegetables that contain lactic acid, yoghurt, buttermilk, and suchlike, have the same effect again: the saliva becomes too acid for the ptyalin to fulfil its digestive function.

While on this subject we should also mention sauces that include yoghurt, vinegar, cider vinegar or lemon juice. Ready-made proprietary sauces and gravies (ketchup, curry sauces, garlic dressing, mustard dressing, and so forth) are invariably highly acidic because of the preservatives they also contain. Commercial sauces of this kind have a pH value between 2.9 and 3.6. Because we generally pile on a lot of sauce, these delicious dressings interfere with the digestion if they are eaten together with potatoes or cereal dishes – yet they can be used with vegetable meals.

Sauerkraut and vegetables containing lactic acid may be combined with other vegetables, but should not be put together with potatoes, rice, buckwheat, bread or other farinaceous foods. Pickled herring (rollmop) with chips/French fries is another bad combination because the vinegar in which the herring has been pickled is still very much in evidence, if only in the background. The same applies to the liquid in which sweet-sour gherkins or cocktail onions are preserved, both of them thoroughly bathed in what is at least partly vinegar.

Many drinks are highly acidic. Cola, for instance, is especially so, with a pH value of 1.9. Soft drinks, coffee and all alcoholic drinks including wines, beers and spirits, greatly affect the degree of acidity of the saliva.

The old school of food combining was under the misapprehension that sugar started to ferment in the stomach if ptyalin was eliminated. But in a combination of starch and acid, there is no possibility of fermentation in the stomach: any problem that does occur with fermentation crops up in the intestines. It is there that the insufficiently digested starch quite likely to be present with such a combination begins to ferment, yet again causing distension of the intestines (bloating) through gas.

Examples of starch-acid combinations include:

bread and tomatoes
bread and apple
spaghetti with tomato sauce
rice with pickled vegetables/vegetables containing lactic acid
potatoes in vinaigrette
pickled herring/rollmop with chips/French fries
sourdough bread
sauerkraut and mashed potatoes
potatoes and sweet-sour gherkins

Acidic drinks include:

cola
soft drinks
coffee
wine
beer/lager
fruit juice (including tomato juice)

Edible oil has a pH value of about 4.5, which means that dressings made of oil or mayonnaise to which a little lemon juice or vinegar has been added have an even higher degree of acidity. If we consume these dressings in fairly thrifty proportions, the combination makes for difficult digestion, but to go overboard and use them in quantity is simply inviting serious digestive disruption. Industrially prepared mayonnaise and dressings should never be used in combination with starchy foods.

Combining Protein and Acid

The digestion of protein begins in the stomach under the influence of the enzyme pepsin (in its eight varietal forms). Quite thorough in the environment of the stomach – pepsin operates in an acidic environment of pH value 2–4 – the process nonetheless continues in the duodenum in a more alkaline setting involving the enzymes trypsin and chymotrypsin. Many people think that eating acidic food assists the acidic gastric juice in the stomach. According to Shelton, however, the presence of acids prevents the secretion of gastric juice, so preventing protein from being digested.

Acid inhibits acid (as we have seen earlier), and this obstructs digestion in the stomach. Mind you, this is only logical, because the degree of acidity in the stomach may be altered by the type of food present. The maximum degree of acidity in the stomach may be as high as pH 1.0, but the food that arrives in the stomach can certainly change that. If the food is highly acidic, the degree of acidity remains high, perhaps too high for the pepsin to function. Moreover, with such an acidity present already, the secretion of gastric juice may also be inhibited: not enough may be produced, and protein may remain undigested. The situation may fluctuate between hyperacidity and hypoacidity. Either way, eating acidic food with protein really does the digestive system no favours at all.

With a combination of protein and acid, the digestion of protein is disrupted: the breakdown remains incomplete. Protein residues may stay in the stomach for too long and begin to degrade, which can lead to an unpleasant taste back up in the mouth. The incomplete digestion then further obstructs protein breakdown in the duodenum, and protein residues continue degrading in the intestine.

Mildly acidic foods have no effect on the workings of the stomach: everything said so far refers to highly acidic foods.

High-protein foods in general should not be eaten together with vegetables that contain lactic acid or other acids, sauerkraut, proprietary sauces and gravies, mustard, or any kind of fruit. But there are one or two exceptions: high-protein foods like cheese and nuts can be eaten in combination with acidic fruit and vegetables. How can there be exceptions? Isn't that a contradiction of the principle of food combining? This is where the proportions of the nutrients in the foods come in. Cheese and nuts have a very high proportion of fats in them, often even higher than protein. So effectively, in this situation, it is not so much a combination of protein and acid as fat and acid, and that is a good combination – or it is if just a little cheese or a few nuts are eaten with a much larger amount of acidic fruit or vegetables.

Because high-protein foods contain fat, a combination of protein and acid is less harmful than a combination of starch and acid. The salivary enzyme works best in a mildly acidic environment, and is therefore more susceptible to acids. The enzymes of the stomach require a more acidic environment (pH 2–4), and can consequently only be influenced by strong acids. Exactly how much acid is present is also significant. Acid and fat form a good combination of foods (inasmuch as emulsification occurs), in which a part of the fat is actually absorbed by the acid.

Many people sprinkle cooked fish with a little lemon juice or put a couple of slices of lemon on it. They do this with the intention of improving their digestion of the fat. In truth, the small quantity of lemon juice has absolutely no effect whatever on gastric function. Pickled herring (rollmop) and the vinegar on it, on the other hand, actively obstruct gastric function. The original form of hot dog, at least as purveyed in north-western Europe, consisted of a hot frankfurter and a helping of sauerkraut inside a split roll or bun. Sauerkraut and frankfurter is a protein-acid combination. Another bad combination that has become popular since then is mustard and cheese.

These last examples show that people often extend a bad combination of foods into a worse one – starch-protein-acid, for instance. The entire fast-food culture is based upon totally the wrong ideas of what food is and what it should do. In addition to the combination of protein and starch, a lot of other acidic material is dumped upon it, like ketchup, mayonnaise, vinegary dressings, and so on. These extra items hinder the digestion of both starch and protein.

Examples of protein-acid combinations include:

meat with vegetables that contain lactic acid
rice with curry sauce
chicken with pineapple
cheese with mustard
frankfurter/sausage with sauerkraut
herring pickled in vinegar
fish and cocktail onions pickled in vinegar

Combining Fat and Sugar

A combination of fat and sugar is unfavourable to digestion. Foods rich in fat almost always have a low content of sugar (carbohydrate). Conversely, foods rich in sugar – such as high-sugar fruits – are low in fat; honey is actually fat-free. Nature shows us that fat and sugar do not belong together.

Wherever there is sugar in a food, there is generally also a lot of water. Some nutritionists like to say 'Sugar swims in water', by which they really mean that sugar is easy to digest in the presence of a sufficient quantity of water. The effect of this is that sugar always occurs in low concentration. Fruits comparatively rich in sugar contain huge proportions also of water. Bananas, for example, which are rich in sugar, are no less than 76 per cent water by volume.

Water and fat are opposites. It is clear that fat and sugar do not belong together.

Table 4.1
The fat-sugar ratio in selected foods

ratio	Fat	Su/St	F:Su
brazil nut	67.0 %	2.3 %	29:1
avocado	23.5 %	0.9 %	26:1
green olive	13.3 %	1.5 %	9:1
black olive	35.8 %	4.9 %	7:1
sunflower seed	49.0 %	8.3 %	5.9:1
hazel nut	61.0 %	10.6 %	5.8:1
almond	54.0 %	9.3 %	5.8:1
linseed	35.0 %	6.0 %	5.8:1
cashew nut	42.2 %	30.5 %	1.4:1

The table demonstrates that in general high-fat foods are low in carbohydrates (Su/St), although there are exceptions like cashew nuts; pine nuts (fat–sugar ratio 3:1) are another exception.

The combination is not a common one. Few people choose to put sugar together with mayonnaise or to sweeten a vinegary dressing. In some countries there are sweet mayonnaises and sauces used with vegetable meals – but they do not make for easy digestion. Raisins and nuts are often used as snacks, and even as a major element of diet for some students. Nut spreads are almost always sweetened with honey or sugar in order to create a sweet sandwich filling. Chocolate, sweetened whipped cream, ice cream, marzipan and nougat are all examples of fat-sugar combinations. They do not help the digestion in any way.

If we eat sugar together with high-fat food, the sugar is mixed with the fat. Sugar is easy to digest. Industrial sugars (disaccharides) are broken down into monosaccharides and absorbed into the bloodstream fairly rapidly. Simple sugars do not require digestion at all: they proceed to the stomach where they are bathed in gastric juice and stabilized by it; they are then conveyed to the duodenum before travelling on to be absorbed in the small intestine. The presence of fat slows this process down, however. Fat inhibits the kneading movement of the stomach wall. Sugar that is completely surrounded by fat cannot make contact with the gastric juice, is not stabilized, and all too quickly begins to ferment.

According to Dr Shelton, sweet fruits and nuts comprise a particularly reprehensible combination despite their delightful aroma together. Sweet fruits are of course rich in sugar. He points out that the combination of fat and sugar is a bad one, and states that avocado and sweet fruits are better not eaten together, presumably for the same reason.

It is the proportional content and composition of foods that are the basis of food combining. Fat and sugar – especially sugar in the industrial form – do not go together. Foods that contain a high proportion of fat should not be sweetened.

A much-loved combination of foods is fruit with whipped cream, which at first sight would appear to be a fat-sugar combination. But that is not quite the case. It is in fact more of a fat-acid-sugar combination. And it all depends on the overall quantity and the constituent proportions, and the specific type of fruit. Fruits that have an acid content obviously have a lower sugar content than sweet fruits. And whipped cream may contain 10 per cent or 30 per cent fat, and we may use just a little or a lot of it.

Some people cannot eat bananas with whipped cream. People who have weak digestive systems may also experience problems after eating sweet fruits with whipped cream. The combination is a difficult one for anybody. But acidic fruits with whipped cream should not cause such difficulties.

Examples of fat-sugar combinations include:

olives with bananas
avocado with sweet fruit
nuts and sweet fruit
cheese and jam
sweetened nut spread
chocolate
nougat
marzipan

Combining Protein and Sugar

Protein and sugar form a bad combination that is not actually all that common anyway. High-protein food seldom contains much in the way of carbohydrates. Among meats, only meat deriving from internal organs (non-muscular tissue) contains carbohydrate in the form of glycogen, and then the quantity is minimal. In vegetable foods such as nuts, seeds and pits/pips, the proportion of carbohydrate is similarly very small, although there are exceptions such as cashew nuts, lupin seeds, pine nuts, sesame seeds, and of course leguminous vegetables.

High-protein food on the other hand always contains a lot of fat. And in this sense, the fat-sugar combination and the protein-sugar combination overlap to an extent. If we add sugar to a high-fat food, we are most likely to arrive at a bad protein-sugar combination as well. Avocado is an exception to this because it actually contains very little protein (1.9 per cent by volume). For all that, the avocado is described as a high-protein fruit/vegetable because its protein content is higher than that of other fruit and vegetables, but in comparison with high-protein foods in general, its protein content is very low.

A sweet dessert at the end of a high-protein meal is always a mistake. For some reason, restaurant cuisine seems to pair meat and fish dishes with fruit, apple sauce or a sweet sauce, a combination that does not improve digestion in any way. High-protein meals remain in the stomach for a relatively long time and are difficult to digest: sugar is not digested fast enough in a well-filled stomach, which may very well lead to fermentation.

Examples of protein-sugar combinations include:

meat with a sweet sauce
fish with fruit
meat with apple sauce
a sweet dessert after a protein-rich meal

Other Bad Combinations

So far we have looked at six bad combinations of food, all of which occur fairly frequently. But there are other bad combinations that are more complicated and require special attention. A few of them are dealt with here; others are mentioned only in passing.

Combining protein and protein

In dietetics it is usual to distinguish between animal protein and vegetable protein. In relation to food combining we distinguish between animal protein (meat and fish), lactoprotein (milk and milk products), protein from a chicken's egg, and vegetable protein (nuts, seeds, pits/pips, cereals and leguminous vegetables).

The digestion of protein is extremely complex, particularly in relation to amino acids. Amino acids are the building-blocks of proteins. Some are released into the stomach by the enzyme pepsin (in its eight varietal forms); others are released into the duodenum by the enzymes trypsin and chymotrypsin; and a final sort is released in the intestinal wall by the hydrolyzing enzyme dipeptidase.

The kind of protein involved is also significant. Lactoprotein is retained in the stomach for quite a long time: the enzyme that is secreted by the stomach wall separates the casein from milk, causing the casein to become fibrous and to stay in the stomach, with the result that pepsin has a longer period to act upon it. Protein from meat is digested faster than protein in egg.

The concentration of the protein is also important. Foods that have a low protein content, like fruits and vegetables, are broken down very easily specifically because the quantity of protein is small.

Proteins of the same derivation may be combined freely in food. This means it is quite all right to eat different kinds of meat during one meal, or different kinds of nuts. A cheese dish together with other kinds of cheese is easy to digest because it contains only lactoprotein. But the effect on the body's acid-base balance must also be borne in mind. Too great a quantity of cheese, nuts, meat or egg can still cause digestive problems.

Dr Shelton rightly labels a milk-egg combination as a bad one. Not so very long ago it was the custom to prepare a drink consisting of an egg beaten in a glass of milk and to give it to the ill and the weak 'to give them strength'. Unfortunately, this 'health' drink actively causes digestive difficulties.

In dietetics, considerable attention has been devoted to the protein chain. By combining specific foods it is possible to make up a shortfall of one type of amino acid in one food using the amino acid present in another food. This ought to be a wonderful discovery, and indeed in theory it is, but in practice it only makes for digestive problems. Much of the protein starts to degrade, which is hardly efficient. Moreover, we do not need all those amino acids at the same time anyway.

Examples of protein-protein combinations include:

> bacon and eggs
> cheese and nuts
> egg with milk

egg with nuts
meat with cheese

Combining fat and fat

In dietetics it is usual to distinguish between animal fat and vegetable fat. For convenience, we here distinguish between animal fats (meat and fish), milk fats (butter, whipped cream, full-fat cheese), egg yolk, and vegetable fats. Fats themselves are composed of saturated, unsaturated and poly-unsaturated fatty acids.

The digestion of fat is relatively simple: there should be no problems at all if gallbladder and liver are working well. Fats are found in almost all foods, but can occur in different proportions.

We should try to avoid mixing different kinds of fat at the same time. So it is best to spread margarine on bread. To fry meat in margarine, for example, is to mix animal and vegetable fats. Some say that grilling meat in its own fat improves the digestion.

To date there is no scientific evidence that eating different kinds of fat is unfavourable to the digestive system. At the same time we do know that no extra fat should be added to a food already rich in fat, for a disproportionate quantity of fat in food does cause digestive problems. The digestive system is simply not capable of processing a lot of fat all at one time, for reasons of capacity rather than anything else, including combination. The disadvantages of a diet that contains too much fat are well known.

Combining protein, fat and fat

The combination of protein and fat is a natural one. All high-protein foods contain fat. The protein remains the dominant nutrient because of its crucial influence on the digestion. But to add fat to a high-protein food is to end up with a protein-fat-fat combination – the addition of single and concentrated fats such as edible oil, margarine and animal fats (beef dripping, lard) to high-protein foods can in particular obstruct digestion.

As we have seen, fat slows down the function of the stomach, which can be a good thing when digesting protein. But if there is too much fat, stomach movement may be over-restricted. Adding fat may make the quantity of fats altogether indigestible. Preparing meat in margarine is composing an unfavourable combination. The decisive factors in relation to this combination are exactly how much fat is added and how strong and healthy the digestive system is.

Combining protein, fat and starch

The combination of protein and starch described earlier is effectively the same thing as a combination of protein, fat and starch. If the amount of fat added is large, problems may result.

Combining protein, fat and sugar

This combination of foods is essentially the same as the combination of protein and sugar plus the combination of fat and sugar both of which were described earlier, for protein is always accompanied by fat.

Combining fat, acid and starch

This combination requires special attention because it is a frequent subject of misunderstanding. Fat and acid is a good combination, as is fat and starch. But what happens if both combinations are used together, when what is eaten is effectively a fat-acid-starch combination? The proportion of acid is the crucial factor. If the quantity of acid is minimal – a few drops of lemon juice or wine vinegar, perhaps, in mayonnaise or in an oil-based salad dressing – it can be ignored. But lashings of acidic sauce on top of starch-rich food is asking for real trouble. Ready-made shop-bought sauces tend to be extremely acidic and go very badly with starchy meals. The acid makes the degree of acidity in the food even higher, altogether eliminating the effect of the enzyme ptyalin in the mouth.

Combining protein, fat, starch and acid

This is an execrable combination, of course, but it is one that in advanced countries is consumed every day in such traditional dishes as meat with potatoes and acidic gravy, or chicken and rice in curry sauce. Four out of five nutrients are present in dominant form. That can happen even in an ordinary food like cake: certainly ordinary cakes or pastries may contain four dominants – protein, fat, sugar and starch. In a cake decorated with whipped cream there may even be five dominants – protein, fat, starch, sugar, and fat again (the whipped cream).

Without doubt, the worst example of a bad combination of foods in one single dish must be muesli. No other dish contains so many combinatory incompatibles. Its ingredients are nuts, oat flakes, raisins, honey, milk and fruit, thus comprising the following nutritional elements: protein (nuts) + protein (milk) + starch (oat flakes) + sugar (honey and raisins) + fat (nuts)

+ acids (in the fruit), or, as we might more graphically express it in symbols, P + P + St + Su + F + A. No fewer than six different nutrients are eaten in nearly equal proportions. Muesli is a nutritional solecism all by itself. Much better for everybody to take an all-fruit breakfast instead.

GOOD FOOD COMBINATIONS

Looking at the long list of combinations of food that are unfavourable, we may well wonder what combinations of food are actually good. The more we study food combining, the more we might be convinced that there are no combinations left that can be good. Well, there are good combinations of food, but only four of them: protein and fat, fat and starch, fat and acid, and sugar and acid.

The protein-fat combination is found naturally in high-protein foods, but is not useful in putting a menu together.

One further potentially good food combination is that of starch and starch, but it is rarely used.

So, all in all, there are basically three good combinations of food that can be taken into account when putting a menu for a meal together. The best way to forget bad combinations of food is to start applying good ones. Limited as they are, they are enough to allow a great variety of different dishes. This section, like the last and the next, presents its information in terms of combinations of nutrients, but we should look at it also from a practical viewpoint, aware that although the number of nutrient combinations may be small, dozens of foods may be combined. The many delicious recipes detailed in Part II illustrate this very point.

Combining Protein and Fat

As has already been said, this is the natural combination of nutrients in high-protein food: protein and fat belong together, occurring in virtually all foods, although often in very small quantities. The great advantage of fat in nutritional terms is that it slows down the function of the stomach so that the accompanying protein has more digestive time and effort devoted to it.

However, the protein-fat combination is found only in diets that consist solely of one type of food or as part of another combination (as, for example, a combination of protein, fat and starch).

Combining Starch and Fat

Foods that are rich in starch – other than the potato – contain quite a lot of protein (7–12 per cent by volume), although the protein-starch ratio in cereals and potatoes is actually the same. And they are low in fat.

The digestion of starch is extremely complex. Initially, predigestion takes place in the mouth, thanks to the enzyme ptyalin. But ptyalin is much affected by the presence of acids, and fats are by definition fatty acids. In addition, they contain antioxidants that prevent them from becoming rancid. So fats can on the one hand inhibit or even nullify the reaction of the salivary enzyme, even as on the other hand the presence of fat improves the digestion in the stomach by lengthening the process.

The presence of fat slows down the peristaltic motion of the stomach wall. Starch stays in the stomach longer, permitting the enhanced digestion of protein.

Combining starchy and fatty foods is favourable to digestion – provided that the overall degree of acidity in the fat is not too high. It is generally of a pH value of 4.5, which would technically be enough to render the saliva rather acid were it not that the added fat (like butter in a sandwich or on fried spaghetti) contains very little fat in relation to the large quantity of starch, so that the combination has a lower degree of acidity. Starch is, moreover, always prepared with water, which dilutes the acid and thus gives a higher (more alkaline) pH value.

The combination of starch and fat is in this way critical to predigestion, because the permitted level of acidity is easily exceeded. If that is something of a disadvantage, it is more than made up for by the favourable influence fat has in the stomach on the digestion of protein. The combination is undoubtedly a good combination on the whole.

Examples of starch-fat combinations include:

bread and butter
bread with avocado
spaghetti and butter
potatoes in an oil dressing
rice cooked in oil
mashed potatoes with home-made mayonnaise
chips/French fries (which are potatoes with fat)

Combining Fat and Acid

This passes for a good combination, although there are conditions. Fat that is used in concentrated form (as in deep-frying, or as beef dripping, coconut oil, or household frying or table oil) is difficult to digest. All concentrated foods, especially in isolation, are difficult to digest. So fats should be used only in restricted quantities.

Sugar can be converted to fat, and there is therefore never any shortage of fat in the body. Acid has a useful effect on fat which, through its agency, becomes emulsified, virtually dissolving the fat and making it easier to digest. A small quantity of lemon juice, wine vinegar or ordinary vinegar can make fat lighter still to digest, and indeed mayonnaise or an oil-based dressing may be almost indigestible without the addition of some such acid. The fat may otherwise remain in the stomach for too long, particularly in people whose digestive systems are not in good health, causing an unpleasant sensation. Drinking a glass of lukewarm water mixed with a little lemon juice should bring immediate relief in these circumstances. Anything described as a vinaigrette usually contains wine vinegar.

Dressings and mayonnaise combine rather well with vegetable meals. Because of their high acid content, however, they should not be put together with high-protein foods, and especially not with foods that are rich in starch. Avocado is best sprinkled or mixed with lemon juice, an ideal constituent of a vegetable meal. If there is no lemon juice available, avocado can be put on bread.

We should always be careful when eating acid and starch together: the limits of digestibility are individual to every person.

As we have seen, nuts or cheese eaten together with acidic fruit represents a fat-acid combination. Fruit is low in protein, so the proportions of fat and acid are not influenced by it, and the acid in the fruit duly emulsifies the fat in the cheese or nuts. Nuts or cheese can also be eaten together with such acid fruits as tomatoes and rhubarb, or with vegetables that contain lactic acid, although the acid limit is exceeded all too easily. Too much acid makes the digestion of protein difficult.

But in general, fat and acid make a good combination. What should be avoided is an addition of acid to the fat in a quantity that makes for a more than merely light emulsifying process, by which the level of acid becomes so high that the food can no longer be combined with starch-rich foods or even high-protein foods (compare the protein-acid and starch-acid combinations).

Examples of fat-acid combinations include:

avocado with lemon juice
an oil-based dressing with wine vinegar
fatty fish with lemon juice
nuts and acidic fruit
cheese and acidic fruit
cheese and tomato

Combining Sugar and Acid

Nobody has ever really considered this combination before. It used to be thought that sugar fermented in the stomach because the salivary enzyme ptyalin was destroyed by gastric juice there. Modern knowledge of the physiology of digestion, and the practical experience of thousands of patients, have proved something entirely different. The digestion of starch that begins in the mouth is temporarily halted in the stomach, where the sugars are stabilized. But the gastric acid does not only stabilize the sugars, it also has protective and bactericidal properties. Any fermentation that does occur is not as a result of the destruction of ptyalin but of the presence of unstabilized sugars which have not made contact with the gastric acid, in turn preventing the ptyalin from continuing its reaction. The upper part of the stomach (its fundus and corpus) acts as a storage chamber. In a well-filled stomach, the food in the middle of this chamber does not touch the wall and starts to ferment – after all, it is warm and humid in the stomach.

This contention is completely contrary to the one propounded by the good doctors Hay and Shelton. Nonetheless, it is striking that Dr Shelton considers yoghurt with honey a good combination, as he does yoghurt with sweet fruit, sugar, or other sweet food. For these are all sugar-acid combinations. On the other hand, he comes down strongly against combining sweet and acidic fruits – a point of view that is not consistent with his favouring the yoghurt and honey combination, for that combination is identical in terms of the nutritional elements. He himself admits he cannot explain this. So, contrary to Dr Shelton's assertion, the combination of sweet and acid fruits is good.

Fruit represents a natural sugar-acid combination, and such harmonious combinations do not have much effect on digestion. There is nothing in modern science to contradict this. We can eat lightly acidic, semi-acidic and acidic fruits together without any digestive problems. If any combination does turn out to be more difficult than others, it is a problem of the individual digestive system and not a problem linked to the combination.

Examples of sugar-acid combinations include:

yoghurt with honey
yoghurt and sweet fruit
buttermilk with sugar
sweet fruit and acidic fruit
sauerkraut with raisins
sweet-and-sour sauce

Combining Starch and Starch

It has been asked whether it is healthy to eat two kinds of starch during one meal. Dr Shelton, discussing the matter, stated that nutritionists recommend only one form of starch per meal, not because there is anything particularly indigestible about such nutrients but because eating two or more starch-rich foods during one meal almost inevitably means overeating. He therefore suggested that everybody, and especially those who were ill, should restrict themselves to only one form of starch per meal.

Starch is always of vegetable origin and belongs to the group of substances known as polysaccharides. The composition of starch can vary, so that one form is different from another – there is, for example, a clear difference between potato starch and cereal starch. Modern research has confirmed Dr Shelton's view that eating different kinds of starch together does not cause digestive problems. In the type of bread that contains five different types of grain, for example, five different types of grain starch are mixed. Mixing grain starch and soya flour is slightly more problematical, however: it leads to an increased proportion of protein, and it is that which causes the digestive difficulty.

Dr Shelton's warning about overeating is apposite enough, but the danger of overeating naturally exists even when only one form of starch is being consumed. Starch is slow to break down into its constituent sugars. So how hungry we feel when eating starch is based not so much on the blood sugar level but on the physical pressure of food against the stomach wall: we go on eating until our stomach feels full – we do not stop after eating one sandwich or one pancake. Too much starch, in addition, disrupts the body's acid-base balance which can thus also cause digestive difficulties. It is remarkable that Dr Shelton said absolutely nothing about this aspect of the combination, whereas Dr Hay made it the basis for his argument in favour of keeping starch and protein separated. In effect, Dr Shelton probably took it into account anyway, if perhaps unconsciously. He recounts that for more than fifty years previously nutritionists had been used to helping themselves to a liberal serving of vegetable salad together with a meal rich in starch, the salad always piled high on the plate and consisting of fresh, raw vegetables.

The combination of starch and starch is a good one. Dr Shelton was speaking more of quantities than of constituent nutrients in combination. Like Dr Shelton, I recommend a diet low in starch for people who are ill as well as for healthy people.

It must be admitted, though, that starch-starch combinations are comparatively rare in any case. There is nothing unwholesome about them, but people seldom eat sandwiches with potatoes, for instance. It is doubtful whether anyone has ever considered baking a potato cake. One frequently found form of starch-starch combination is the potato croquette, in which a mashed potato roll is covered in breadcrumbs and deep-fried, but this is really a starch-starch-fat combination.

Buffet dishes or snacks in a restaurant are often based on farinaceous ingredients. Such dishes include potato salad, potato croquettes, miniature pizzas or pizza-bits, different kinds of sandwiches, and savoury biscuits with different toppings. It is not wrong to have several of these attractive little things on our plate.

Examples of starch-starch combinations include:

potato croquette
potato with a miniature pizza
different kinds of pasta
bread made of different grains
different kinds of bread or rolls

PROBLEMATICAL COMBINATIONS

After reading this far, it may well seem that there are a few good combinations of foods and a lot of bad ones. But nothing on the subject of food can ever be quite so clear-cut. Every type of food has a different composition. By combining foods, the proportions of nutrients in them are changed for the better or the worse. The idea of a limit of tolerance (the level at which a food becomes simply indigestible) has been mentioned once or twice. Yet it is not easy to define that limit in relation to specific combinations, although of course some foods should never be combined. There are, after all, also combinations that people can tolerate if they have a strong enough digestive system.

The protein-starch combination is a bad one. An example is the ubiquitous slice of bread and cheese. But there is a great difference between a sandwich with a thick slice of cheese and the same sandwich with a thin slice. There is a similar difference between a sandwich with a lot of butter or margarine and the same sandwich with only a little. A cheese sandwich is easier to digest if salad is added, rather than mustard. Whether we eat one sandwich or a whole pile of sandwiches also makes a considerable difference. So many factors have a crucial influence on digestion.

It should be made clear from the outset, however, that a bad combination can never be transformed into a good one. All that can be done with a bad combination is to try to improve it by restoring the acid-base balance somehow (perhaps by adding salad) or by limiting the quantity consumed.

So, provided our digestive systems are functioning reasonably well, we can improve on the combinations that in this book are described as difficult or problematical. Those people whose digestive system is in poor health should restrict themselves to the good combinations of food because they cannot tolerate the least deviation.

Do not be too quick to believe that you are one of the exceptions who can digest everything and anything. Acid indigestion, a stomach bloated with food and wind, flatulence, diarrhoea or constipation – all are clear symptoms of digestive difficulty even when you are not ill.

It is not possible to describe basic problematical combinations in the way we did with the bad and the good combinations. This section deals with a number of different types of food that are difficult (but not impossible) to digest when used as the sole constituent of a diet, or that can cause problems when combined with other foods.

The list is by no means exhaustive.

Combining protein with foods low in starch

Protein and starch form a bad combination. There are types of food that contain only minimal starch, but even this tiny quantity can cause serious problems in those who have a weak digestive system (although it does not cause problems in healthy systems). What we are talking about here are vegetables that have a starch content of around and slightly more than 4 per cent; a content of less than 4 per cent is negligible.

Examples include:

high-protein foods with pumpkin
                       winter radish
                       kohlrabi
                       French beans
                       Jerusalem artichoke

Combining protein with mildly acidic or semi-acidic fruit

As we have seen, protein with acidic fruit is a bad combination unless the fat present is dominant (as it is, for instance, in the combination of nuts or cheese with acidic fruit). For people with a sensitive digestive system, even the acid in a mildly acidic fruit may cause problems; moreover, this combination very much depends on individual digestive reaction.

Combining fruit and vegetables

Fruit and vegetables are almost nutritional opposites. Fruits are acidic, vegetables are usually not. Fruits contain a lot of sugar, most vegetables contain only a trace. Eating fruit and vegetables together can cause digestive problems. As far as possible, they should be eaten separately – and vegetable juice counts as vegetables in this connection. Nonetheless, as has been stated earlier, this combination is not a bad one, just a difficult one.

Leguminous vegetables

Legumes are always difficult to digest. But their digestion can be improved by combining them with other types of vegetables, which has the effect of restoring the acid-base balance. Even in the most favourable circumstances, however, every dish that contains leguminous vegetables remains a difficult combination. The same applies to soya products, with the exception of tofu (soybean curd).

Milk

Milk does not take to being combined with other foods easily; it is a drink that pretty well has to be used on its own. With fruit or vegetables, milk forms a problematical combination.

CHAPTER 5

FRUIT AND VEGETABLES

The fruits are among the finest and best of all foods. Nothing is more enjoyable to eat than a succulent, chunky apple, a delicious ripe banana, a carefully compiled basket of fruits, a creamy mellow avocado, or the healthy heart-warming juiciness of a sweet grape. The epitome of tastiness is a peach that has attained perfect ripeness. Fruits are the peak of pleasure to the sense of taste, a treasure-store of miraculous food. With their extravagant mixture of rare scents, their exciting aroma, and their eyecatching colours, fruits remain an ever-fresh inspiration to the appetite.

But fruits are more than a mere delight to the eye, nose and mouth: they are exquisite collections of pure, rich, watery food constituents. Few of them contain much in the way of protein, with the exception of the avocado and the olive, but they contain sugars to make one's mouth water, they are drenched in fragrant streams of acids, and they are full of minerals and vitamins. Like nuts, these foods are just ideal for the naturally fruit-eating animal that is the human being.

Eating fruit provides us with an exceptionally intense pleasure. Mother Nature scented fruits in such a way as to give us the maximum of gratification. Nothing could be more satisfying to the taste-buds. We have every reason to eat the foods with which Mother Nature tempts us so compellingly, and to enjoy such pleasures from the fruits. She has filled with such pure, rich and beneficent nutrients.

Adapted from Dr Herbert M. Shelton: *Food Combining . . . Made Easy*,
San Antonio, Texas, 1951.

Dr Shelton has described fruit splendidly. It is remarkable that whereas many people shower praise upon fruits, berries and nuts, traditional cuisine tends to look down on fruit. Fruits have a low calorific value, and contain little protein and fat – and are therefore regarded as inferior. Contemporary cookery books cite fruits as good sources of vitamins and minerals, but then go on to warn of the dangers of eating too much of them. The authors suggest that one or two fruits per day is more than sufficient. All these years

I have been trying to have fruit accepted as the sustaining nourishment it is, while my colleagues in traditional dietetics have been reluctant to see it as any such thing.

In alimentary medicine, fruit is very often the villain. Digestive problems, wind caused by fermentation, and other stomach and intestinal problems are frequently blamed on fruit. Fruit is at the top of the list of forbidden foods.

Many of the problems listed above may well have something to do with the consumption of fruit, but people forget that fruit is eaten in the wrong way. It is cooked, or eaten in the form of a sauce, a jelly or a jam. It is virtually always treated as a dessert. It is often eaten when unripe. And it is frequently combined with other foods unsuited to it.

Like berries and the type of fruit and vegetables known as gourds (which include melons), fruit is difficult to combine with other foods. The nutrients in fruit that are decisive in food combining are sugar and acids: fruit is a natural sugar-acid combination. But that is why fruit combines badly: acids do not combine with starch or protein, sugars do not combine with starch, protein or fat. So five combinations are not possible.

Fruits, including berries and melons, cannot be combined with bread, cereal dishes, pasta, meat or fish. Avocado and olives, which are both extremely rich in fat, may be combined with starch, but not with fruits that are rich in sugar.

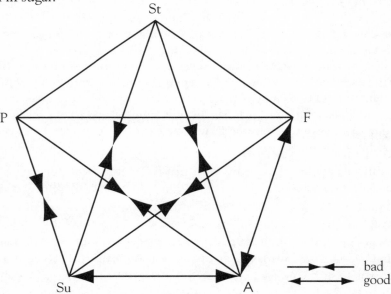

This pentagon shows the good and bad combinations of sugar and acid.

A jam sandwich – a sugar-starch combination – is a bad combination. A banana sandwich, which is another popular confection, is also extremely inadvisable because of the inherent sugar-starch and starch-acid combinations. It is forever being overlooked that, for all its sweet taste, a banana is as acidic as a tomato. The high sugar content masks the acidic taste. The tomato contains only 3 per cent sugar, which is why the acids in it are clearly discerned.

As far as possible, we should eat fruit as a separate dish or meal, and not combine it with other foods. As a meal in itself, or as a casual snack, fruit can be digested smoothly and easily. If someone still experiences digestive difficulties, the cause could well be something different – a change of working shifts, for example. When shifts are changed, people tend to eat too much and too fast. Or snatching food between shifts, a person may stuff his or her stomach with fruit (or indeed with any food). I have often been surprised by the large quantities of fruit that some people seem to eat per meal. They may think they know all about fruit-eating, but they really understand little about fruit diets.

Fruit should be eaten slowly, and in small amounts. The fruit should be allowed to melt in the mouth so that the sugars can be released and be absorbed into the bloodstream. Sugar in the bloodstream affects the saturation centre in the hypothalamus of the brain: our appetite is satisfied relatively quickly, and we do not feel obliged to eat more than a small quantity. That is the way to obtain perfect digestion. If we eat too fast, we swallow large lumps of fruit that the stomach cannot properly break down. This is how undigested residues come to ferment in the intestines.

Is it possible to eat too much fruit? It certainly is. A person who does so has to eliminate excessive quantities of potassium through the kidneys, which means an annoying frequency and urgency in urination and burdensome pressure on the kidneys and the bladder. Years of experience with cancer patients on a strict fruit diet (the Dries cancer diet) have taught me that cancer patients can get by with relatively little fruit per day as soon as they switch over to a fruit-only diet. The daily intake is not more than 1.5 kilograms (3.3 pounds), and blood tests show that there are no nutritional deficiencies.

Fresh fruit juice is equal to fruit in every way, although digestion is actually a lot easier because everything has been reduced to liquid even before reaching the mouth. Fruit juice can be compared with breast-feeding (nursing). The supposition that fruit juice contains no roughage (dietary fibre) is inaccurate, for fruit juice is merely the liquidized form of the whole food.

(Mother's milk does not contain roughage as such either, but the baby still has bowel movements.)

FRUIT COMBINATIONS

Dr Shelton distinguished between sweet, semi-acidic and acidic fruits. I am not aware of what he based this division upon, but it may well have been the direct tastes of the fruits. Unhappily, the division does not work, and all his contentions about food combining in relation to fruits have therefore to be ignored. It is just not the case that sweet fruit (fruit with few acids and plenty of sugar) may not be combined with acidic fruit (fruit with plenty of acids and comparatively little sugar).

Sugar and acid form a good combination, as we have already seen. All fruit contains sugar and acid, one more than the other, so putting combinations of fruit together does not change anything. Mixing sweet fruit with acidic fruit means that what is digested might as well be semi-acidic fruit. Of course the effect is not always averaged out quite so evenly, but any difference is so small as not to influence digestion.

Shelton stated that from providing meals to the ill he discovered that it was best to serve sweet fruit and acidic fruit as separate meals. His grouping of specific fruits into sweet, semi-acidic and acidic is 80 per cent inaccurate in any case. He considers pineapple to be an acidic fruit, for instance, when it is in fact a sweet fruit. There is no scientific reason why sweet and acidic fruits should not be combined. The stabilization of sugars in the sweet fruit is totally accounted for by the acids in the acidic fruit. Many people whom I know to have been familiar with the principle of food combining for years have told me that never once have they tried to avoid combining all types of fruit, and that they have never had any problems because of it. They are quite used to eating all kinds of fruit together.

I gave a banana mixed with lemon juice to some people whom I knew had digestive problems. The reaction was unanimous: never had they eaten a banana that digested so comfortably. Shelton was right in saying that there are ill people who cannot tolerate certain combinations of foods, but that applies also to some healthy people and equates with an individual reaction that has nothing to do with the combination involved.

The amount of fruit per meal should not exceed 500–600 grams (1–1¼ pounds). This puts no pressure on the stomach. To live only on fruit requires several meals a day, and in most cases other fruits like nuts are necessary in order to ensure the full complement of nutrients. People whose digestive systems are weak benefit from eating only one kind of fruit, despite the possibilities of food combining. Eating solely one type of food makes for the most relaxed digestion, and technically, nothing is better than such a diet. People whose digestive systems are healthier can combine a diet like this with other fruits that they know they tolerate well. Ordinarily healthy people should not experience any problems except in relation to the types of fruit they personally do not tolerate well.

Fruit can be combined with fruit without qualms: it is not necessary to take the acid or sugar content into account at all.

OTHER POTENTIAL COMBINATIONS

Fruit, and especially sweet fruit, goes well together with acidic foods like yoghurt, buttermilk, sour cream and even sauerkraut. Acidic fruits may be combined with fatty foods such as full-fat curd cheese, hard and semi-hard cheeses, nuts, seeds and pips rich in fat. Fruit with unsweetened whipped cream is also a good combination because the acid is then the dominant nutrient. Even the 'sweet' banana has a pH value of 3.8, which makes it just as acidic as a tomato. People whose digestive systems are sensitive may experience difficulties when they eat large quantities of sweet fruit together with whipped cream that is rich in fat.

Sweet fruit and whipped cream in turn combined with foods rich in starch (such as a cake or pastry) represents a bad combination for anyone.

GOURDS

Gourds are types of fruit and vegetables that come from climbing plants. Only the honeydew melon and the Spanish yellow melon have any genuine sugar content, the others contain mere traces of carbohydrates. Unlike other fruits, therefore, they are mildly acidic and should be considered a separate group of foods in connection with food combining.

Other than the honeydew and the yellow melon, melons are almost 94 per cent water: they are otherwise made up of 1 per cent protein, 0.2 per cent fat and 5.3 per cent carbohydrates. In terms of energy melon supplies only 25 kilocalories per 100 grams (104.6 kilojoules per 100 grams). Dr Shelton advises people to eat melon on its own.

The honeydew and the yellow melon contain sugar, however, and can be combined with other fruits.

The vegetable gourds – such as pumpkin, courgettes, cucumber, gherkins and aubergine – can be combined with other (non-leguminous) vegetables because they are similar in composition to them.

VEGETABLES

The composition of vegetables is completely different from that of fruit, which is why vegetables and fruit should never be eaten together: it is a difficult or problematical combination.

The major difference between vegetables and fruit lies in the relative proportions of protein, carbohydrates and acids. Fruits have a fairly high content of sugar and acid, but are low in protein. Vegetables are low in sugar and contain little by way of acids, but they are slightly richer in protein: the lower their sugar content, the more fruit acids they contain. Acids and sugars have a reciprocal relationship.

With the exception of the tomato (if it may be considered a vegetable), vegetables do not contain much acid – their pH value is around 5.2–6.6, which makes them only mildly acidic. This is why they may be combined readily with protein and starch. (Dr Hay regarded vegetables as neutral in relation to protein and starch.)

The actual structure of vegetables is generally harder, more solid, than that of fruit, and that is one reason they are more difficult to digest. The problem may be solved by the addition of mayonnaise or an oil-based dressing. This causes the vegetables to remain longer in the stomach so that digestion is given extra time. Raw vegetables with no dressing are problematical for the digestion. Humans are not natural herbivores and we should ensure that vegetables always receive a minimum of preparation.

In terms of food combining, there is no difference between raw and cooked vegetables.

CHAPTER 6

HOW TO COMBINE FOOD
CORRECTLY

To break old habits it is often necessary to sever the ties that have contributed to the formation of those habits and that reinforce them. A change of lifestyle and environment is frequently the best way of cutting oneself free from whatever it was that first started one off on unsuitable mental and physical routines, and from the influences that since then have kept one in their thrall. A determinedly resolute person should be able to regard such potentially injurious elements of his or her daily existence as obstacles that can be overcome. But it is something of a pity that there are so few determinedly resolute people around.

> Adapted from Dr Herbert M. Shelton: *Food Combining . . . Made Easy*,
> San Antonio, Texas, 1951.

I hope that you are by now convinced of the benefits of food combining. The principle of sticking to good combinations of food that I have described is scientifically sound, and corresponds to present-day knowledge of the physiology of digestion. If you have any remaining doubts, I ask you just to try it out for yourself. Have one meal that accords with the theory of food combining, and another meal in the way you are accustomed to. You should notice a great difference.

Good food combining renders digestion easy and comfortable both after and during the actual eating. When the stomach is full, it expands slightly, but there is no heavy feeling. On the contrary, with good food combining the stomach empties faster and uses less energy. Thousands of people already enjoy the advantages of food combining. For many of them it has led to their regaining health or throwing off disease.

One obvious question arises: How can we learn to combine foods correctly? How can we put this wonderful theory into daily practice? It may look a little complicated, but really it is not difficult at all. The starting-point is, as ever, the familiar pentagon on which the five nutrients are displayed with their good and bad relationships in combination. It is the dominant nutrient in any food that determines whether or not the food may be combined with another food.

It all comes down to having a fair grasp of the five groups. If I were to ask you which group jelly, jam, honey or syrup belonged to, you would know the answer immediately: sugar. If I were to ask you to list several high-protein foods, you would be able to do so easily, I'm sure. Other groupings may be slightly more obscure. Is fruit grouped with the sugars or with the acids? Fruit, of course, contains both sugars and acids. If we are wondering about a fruit that is rich in sugar, we have to take the sugar into account. When thinking of fruits in combination with other foods, we have to take account of both the sugar and the acid content.

In addition to the five nutrients, there are some forms of food that have very little effect on food combining. Dr Hay pointed out that (non-leguminous) vegetables have something of a neutral character, for example. With the exception of the tomato (if that is a vegetable at all), vegetables can be combined with both protein and starch. I have tended to avoid using the word 'neutral' in this sense of 'inert', for fear that it might be confused with neutrality between acidity and alkalinity. To me, a neutral food would have a pH value of 7 – and such foods do not exist. Fresh milk and eggs, however, come close to having a neutral value.

Vegetables contain a lot of water but not much carbohydrate, acid or fat, and very little protein. The protein content is actually higher than that of fruit, but it is very low in comparison with the protein content of high-protein foods. If we add vegetables to other foods, the overall proportions of nutrients barely change. This is why vegetables are easy to combine with just about everything – although there are exceptions, such as vegetables with sugar. If vegetables are combined with sugar, the sugar content, which is always very low in vegetables, is proportionately increased by enough to alter the nutrient ratio. So sugar or honey should never be eaten with raw vegetables. Acids go well with vegetables. But because fruit contains acids and sugar, fruit together with vegetables is a combination that is problematical for the digestion.

Another form of food that combines well with other foods is the mushroom. It contains remarkably little acid (its pH value is 6.4), hardly any fat and carbohydrates, and relatively little protein (2.7 per cent by volume). The water content is extremely high (94 per cent), and in energy it produces only 15 kilocalories per 100 grams (62.8 kilojoules per 100 grams). Combining mushrooms with other foods has very little effect at all on overall nutrient proportions. Although in theory there can be no bad combination involving mushrooms, they are not suitable for putting together with absolutely every-thing. Their aroma is also significant. It is uncommon to eat mushrooms with nuts, seeds or pits/pips, or with sugar, fruit, yoghurt or milk – although a milk or yoghurt sauce incorporating mushrooms is standard enough. All fungi are comparable with mushrooms; only the truffle has rather more in the way of protein (5 per cent).

In terms of its composition, cow's milk is more or less comparable with vegetables. It contains plenty of water, but little protein, fat, carbohydrate and acid. Milk is a whole food in liquid form. It can be combined only with acidic foods: it readily increases in acidity, so improving digestion, and that is why acidic foods are the only good form of combination with it. Milk with fat, milk with fruit, or milk with vegetables are to be regarded as problematical combinations.

Water-melon is rich in water and low in nutrients, but for all that is not easy to combine. All melons are best eaten separately. Water-melon can, however, be eaten in small quantities mixed with other fruit.

LEARNING TO EVALUATE

There are two methods of finding out about specific combinations of food. A comprehensive table showing the names of particular foods grouped according to the dominant nutrient in each is to be found on page 99. Alter-natively, it is not difficult to judge for oneself whether a combination is favourable or not by finding out what the ingredients are in the proposed meal, listing them, and checking what group or groups of nutrients they should be classified with, and in what proportion. Then, reference to the pentagon or to the abbreviated diagram below should provide enough infor-mation about whether the combination is good or bad.

This diagram overleaf presents a schema slightly different from the pentagon's. Protein can be combined with protein if it is of the same form; different kinds of protein should not be combined, and that is why there are two possibilities represented on the diagram. Similarly, fat combines easily with fat. It is also possible to mix different kinds of fat, although that is unusual. But if fat is added to foods that are already rich in fat, the overall proportion of fat may be too large, resulting in a problematical combination. Starch with starch is a good combination, as is the combination of different kinds of sugar or different kinds of acids.

Looking at the composition of a dish or a menu, we should be able sooner or later to analyse whether it represents a good, bad, or problematical

	P	F	Su	St	A
A	–	✓	✓	–	✓
St	–	✓	–	✓	–
Su	–	–	✓	–	✓
F	–	✓ ✕	–	✓	✓
P	✓ –	–	–	–	–

✓ good combination
– bad combination
✕ difficult or problematical combination

Abbreviated diagram of food combinations.

combination, based on that data. But to be correct in detail is a possibility really restricted to nutritional experts who have to apply such knowledge in order to prescribe diets for the ill (diet therapy). In general, we should let intuition and instinct judge. It should be possible to come to a conclusion about the nature of a combination by optical observation. Statistics and measurements are useful at first in order to develop that intuition and instinct, to know what to look for. But after a while, we should have a very good idea at sight of what can and cannot be combined.

Here are two examples of how initial calculations might turn out.

Example A

Foods	P (%)	F (%)	St (%)
200 g (7 oz) potatoes	2.0	0.1	15.4
60 g (2 oz) mushrooms	2.7	0.3	–
150 g (5 oz) vegetables	1.5	0.3	–
12 g (½ oz) oil (as dressing)	–	100	–
TOTAL	1.9	3.1	7.3

ratios: P:St 1:3.8
        F:St 1:2.4

Example B

Foods	P (%)	F (%)	St (%)
200 g (7 oz) potatoes	2.0	0.1	15.4
150 g (5 oz) beef	19.0	4.5	–
150 g (5 oz) vegetables	1.5	0.3	–
12 g (½ oz) butter (in frying)	–	100	–
TOTAL	6.8	3.8	6.0

ratios: P:St 1:0.9 (more protein than starch)
F:St 1:1.6

Example A represents a good protein-starch combination in which the fat-starch ratio is also favourable. But in Example B, protein and starch are both dominant and the fat-starch ratio is less favourable. It is a bad combination.

This is how to evaluate a menu.

It should be emphasized once again that it is the overall proportions of the nutrients in the foods which are the key to food combining. Protein together with starch is a bad combination, but it is the amount of protein and the amount of starch that determine if a combination is good, bad, or problematical. All foods, even farinaceous foods, contain protein. Combination is nonetheless possible, as long as permissible limits are not exceeded. What those permissible limits are, exactly, can in theory be determined by analytical calculations, but in practice it is not that simple because several other factors also influence matters – such factors as a healthy acid-base balance, the actual quantity of food consumed, how well the food is chewed, the overall health and efficiency of the digestive system, and so forth.

In evaluating a combination of foods, we start by assessing the capacity of the nutrients to combine in terms of their overall quantities. We need to know the quantities of nutrients because they determine the proportions of the nutrients in relation to each other and to the physical quantity of the food. Remember, the proportions of the nutrients and the overall quantity of food are two separate elements that influence the digestive character of the combination. A favourable nutrient ratio is essential. If the protein-starch ratio of a combination of foods is 1:5, the combination is good. But if the protein-starch ratio is 1:1, the combination is bad. If a dish contains 35 grams of protein and 35 grams of starch, digestion will be very difficult. If a dish consists of 3 grams of protein and 3 grams of starch, digestion should be virtually smooth even though the ratio is the same. We must always keep a close eye on both the nutrient proportions and the quantities.

We evaluate the combination in each dish, and afterwards the overall combination of the meal. In a dish different foods are put together. They should be chosen to combine well together. And indeed, the whole menu should be composed of dishes that combine well together – it is a waste of time, after all, to prepare dishes that are each of a good combination if together they react badly with one another. We should not serve a high-protein starter if the main course is rich in starch. Even though the stomach fills itself in layers from the outside in, and gastric digestion follows the same process, the whole of the stomach contents have to be taken into account: it is the composition of those entire contents that are decisive for good food combining. A meal consists of one or more dishes, but should always be considered as a whole. There is no harm at all in eating several dishes consecutively as long as they do not disrupt the overall combination.

For many, if not most, people, breakfast and supper consist of one dish. It is strange, then, that when one travels, the breakfast that is served (in hotels and motels) is much more elaborate. In some tourist hotels, the breakfast buffet is an entire selection of different foods. From that ample provision the right choice has to be made. Do not eat everything you see, but eat what goes well together.

Dinner, on the other hand, although often postponed until the evening, consists of several dishes: starter and/or soup, main course, and dessert. Most people eat one elaborate meal a day. At a dinner or celebratory lunch, there may also be side-dishes. Traditional cooking most commonly makes the main course a combination of protein and starch (such as meat with potatoes, chicken with rice, fish and potato croquettes). According to the principle of food combining, protein and starch should be eaten separately. Meat with ordinary vegetables, or potatoes with the vegetables, would be fine. Vegetarians should also make the choice between a high-protein dish or a dish rich in starch.

The choice of the main course should determine the entire menu. A high-protein main course means that the dominance of protein must be taken into account. The same applies if the main course we choose is rich in starch. Let us have a look at both of these possibilities separately.

If we are planning a high-protein main course, we tend to repeat that combination in the other dishes. A classic example is a meal made up thus: pea soup, followed by Parma ham, the main course of meat, and a dessert of cheese. As a combination of foods with similar nutrient ratios this is an excellent menu, but it is rather too heavy. The acid-base balance would be disturbed, and badly. There is just too much protein. If a menu contains a high-protein dish, we should ensure that other dishes are as light as possible.

Let us improve on this example. The pea soup is replaced by a light vegetable soup. Instead of the ham, there might be raw vegetables, possibly supplemented with a little meat or fish, but only in small amounts. The main dish can stay. But it would be best to cut out the dessert altogether. Such traditional desserts really have no place following high-protein dishes or dishes rich in starch.

All that is needed is a little creativity to produce new desserts.

In a healthy diet, a menu may be regarded as comprising a single gigantic dish divided into different courses. After all, it is eaten in courses, which is a good thing in itself: a meal eaten in several courses is eaten much more slowly and is interrupted by breaks. It is a lot more enjoyable to eat than one gigantic dish.

Soup, apart from high-protein soup, has very little effect on the combination of the dishes that follow it. We now know that the liquid of the soup is filtered off quickly down the 'gastric passage' on the inner curved stomach wall and does not dilute the gastric juice. Only the solids in the soup are left deposited and waiting to be digested. After the soup we should not go straight on to a sweet starter/entrée. There is nothing wrong with having a sweet starter/entrée before having the soup, however. A high-protein meal could be preceded by half a honeydew melon, possibly filled with berries in a suitable sauce. The sugar will digest quickly, and because the sweet starter is eaten first it will also leave the stomach first. Fruit can always be used as a starter. Dr Shelton rightly pointed out that fruit should be eaten before, and not after, a meal.

But the starter has to be matched with the soup as much as possible. It should preferably be a small dish consisting of raw vegetables. If the main course is a high-protein dish, the starter should not be too acidic (like sauerkraut, vegetables containing lactic acid, or sour cream) because acid inhibits acid, as we have seen earlier, and inhibition of the production of gastric acid would be a disaster when we need a lot of gastric acid to digest the high-protein main course. Shelton claims that fatty meat, full-fat cottage cheese and fatty fish form a better combination with acidic foods than meats, cheeses and fish that are low in fat. That is not correct, however. Fat and acid represents a good combination that lightens the digestion of high-fat and high-protein foods. Eating low-fat foods is to miss out on the function of the fat, which is to slow down the gastric peristalsis. High-protein foods that are low in fat are more difficult to digest than those that are rich in fat. By adding acid to low-fat foods we effectively slow gastric motility: that is why acid does not necessarily have to be avoided.

In our discussion of the protein-acid combination it was pointed out that acid should be used in moderation. With foods that are high in protein but low in fat we are allowed to use more acid than with foods that are rich in fat. When we eat high-fat foods, both the fat and the acid slow down the gastric peristalsis. We should also be sure to eat only one form of protein per meal.

If the proposed menu is rich in starch, the procedure is the same. Although sweet and acidic should not be combined with starch, both can precede a meal that is rich in starch. If we eat a sweet starter/entrée first, the sugar is stabilized by the gastric juice in the stomach and goes on fairly rapidly into the duodenum. The sugar has no effect on the starch that is to follow. In the final part of the stomach (the antrum), fermentation is not possible. If we eat an acidic starter/entrée, the acidity of the saliva is increased. But as soon as we start on the dish that is rich in starch, a new type of saliva geared to treat the starchy food is produced.

A menu that contains dishes rich in starch must not also contain high-protein dishes.

It is important that the contents of the stomach are controlled by the one dominant nutrient, whether it is protein, starch or sugar. Fat and acid are highly significant to digestion, but they cannot control the processing by the stomach. Fat is related to protein, acid to sugar.

THE DIAGRAM OF COMBINATIONS

To make things easy for you, here is a diagram of food combinations. They are grouped according to the five nutrients, so making it simple to check up on the principle behind food combining. There is an additional group comprising (non-leguminous) vegetables, mushrooms and milk because these fairly common foods do not fall into any of the other categories.

Using this diagram, everyone can participate in food combining and successfully avoid bad combinations of food. But it is simply not possible to classify all foods in the diagram. That would make the whole thing far too complex. All that is necessary, after all, is a rough and ready working knowledge of the subject, and particularly of foods in their groups. If you wonder what buckwheat can be combined with, for example, look under 'cereals'. Or if you want to know what a soya burger can be combined with, you will find it under 'meat'.

			acids					starch			sugar		fat			protein		
		mushrooms	milk	vegetables	vegetables (lactic acid)	yoghurt – butter milk	tomato	vinegar – mustard	fruits – berries	vegetables rich in starch	potato	cereals – bread – pasta	fruit rich in sugar	sugar – honey	avocado – olive	butter – whipped cream	oil – fat – egg yolk	nuts – seeds – pips	cheese – cottage cheese	meat – fish – poultry
protein	meat – fish – poultry	✓	–	✓	–	–	✓	–	–	✗	–	–	–	–	–	–	–	–	–	■
	cheese – cottage cheese	✓	–	✓	–	✗	✓	–	✓	✗	–	–	–	–	–	–	–	–	■	–
	nuts – seeds – pips	•	–	✓	✓	✗	✓	–	✓	✗	–	–	–	–	–	–	–	■	–	–
fat	oil – fat – egg yolk	✓	✗	✓	✓	✓	✓	✓	✓	✓	✓	✓	✓	✗	–	–	■	–	–	–
	butter – whipped cream	✓	✗	✓	✓	✓	✓	✓	✓	✓	✓	✓	✓	✗	–	■	–	–	–	–
	avocado – olive	✓	–	✓	✓	✓	✓	✓	✓	✓	✓	✓	–	✓	■	–	–	–	–	–
sugar	sugar – honey	–	–	–	–	✓	•	•	✓	✗	–	–	✗	■	✓	✗	✗	–	–	–
	fruit rich in sugar	–	–	–	–	✓	–	✗	✓	✗	–	–	■	✗	–	✓	✓	–	–	–
starch	cereals – bread – pasta	✓	–	✓	–	–	–	–	–	✓	✓	■	–	–	✓	✓	✓	–	–	–
	potato	✓	–	✓	–	–	–	–	–	✓	■	✓	–	–	✓	✓	✓	–	–	–
	vegetables rich in starch	✓	–	✓	✓	✓	✗	✗	✗	■	✓	✓	✗	✗	✓	✓	✓	✗	✗	✗
acids	fruits – berries	–	✗	✗	✗	✓	✗	✓	■	✗	–	–	✓	✓	✓	✓	✓	✓	✓	–
	vinegar – mustard	✓	✗	✓	✗	–	✓	■	✓	✗	–	–	✗	•	✓	✓	✓	–	–	–
	tomato	✓	✗	✓	✓	✓	■	✓	✗	✗	–	–	–	•	✓	✓	✓	✓	✓	✓
	yoghurt – butter milk	•	✓	✓	✓	■	✓	–	✓	✓	–	–	✓	✓	✓	✓	✓	✗	✗	–
	vegetables (lactic acid)	✓	✗	✓	■	✓	✓	✗	✗	✓	–	–	–	–	✓	✓	✓	✓	–	–
	vegetables	✓	✗	■	✓	✓	✓	✓	✗	✓	✓	✓	–	–	✓	✓	✓	✓	✓	✓
	milk	•	■	✗	✗	✓	✗	✗	✗	–	–	–	–	–	–	✗	✗	–	–	–
	mushrooms	■	•	✓	✓	•	✓	✓	–	✓	✓	✓	–	–	✓	✓	✓	•	✓	✓

✓ good combinations ✗ difficult combinations
– bad combinations • good, but not usual

PRACTICAL GUIDELINES

The more you know about food combining, the greater is the urge to set fire to all your cookery books. Not a single cookery book makes any allowance for food combining. But you can keep your cookery books on condition that you rewrite them yourself: choose some of the recipes, and try to adjust them and alter them so that they combine well. It is possible to be very creative with food, and particularly so if the principles of food combining are borne in mind.

To help you find your way around the maze of statistics and measurements that food combining seems initially to be, here are a few practical tips. Of course they represent ideas that have already appeared earlier in this book, but in this section they are intended to be useful reminders.

- Remember that digestion is a complex process. Food combining encourages this process to take place as smoothly and efficiently as possible.
- Not to practise food combining means continuing digestive problems. You may feel something is wrong even while you are still eating. If the food lies heavy on the stomach from the start, the whole process of digestion is very unlikely to be smooth and efficient.
- Acid indigestion, wind in the stomach and intestines, flatulence, breathlessness, obesity and sometimes food allergy can all be caused by combining the wrong types of food.
- Food combining can be applied to any eating pattern. You do not have to be a vegetarian (for example) to benefit from favourable combinations of food.
- Food combining is closely linked with digestion: the better the digestion, the better the body's absorption and metabolism. Good health begins with good digestion.
- The breakdown of food inevitably produces wastes. Food combining ensures that these wastes are limited to a minimum, which means that there is also a higher output. You need less food and get more out of it. It will also cost you less energy to digest a small quantity of food. With fewer waste products, there is less risk of toxic degradation. Toxins are removed more easily, and accumulation should be impossible.
- Digestion takes place in the mouth, the stomach, the duodenum, the small intestine, and the large intestine. Starch is predigested in the mouth thanks to the salivary enzyme ptyalin, which requires a mildly acidic environment. That is why acidic foods (that have a low pH value) should not be combined with foods that are rich in starch.
- Drinking before, during, or after meals does not dilute the gastric juice. The liquid is filtered off quickly down the inner curved wall of the stomach. Acidic drinks like cola, coffee and carbonated spring water render the saliva more acidic, which inhibits the predigestion in the mouth of foods rich in starch. Drinking when the stomach is already full, however, can lead to an unpleasant sensation as the liquid cannot follow its usual rapid course through the stomach, remaining like a bubble at the bottom of the oesophagus or in the top of the stomach.

- Protein undergoes its first digestive process in the stomach under the influence of the enzyme pepsin (in its eight or so varietal forms), which only works in an acidic environment.
- The presence of fat in the duodenum causes the kneading movements of the stomach wall to slow down, with the result that protein is subject to gastric acids for a longer time in the stomach. This demonstrates the natural relationship between fat and protein. If extra fat is added, the stomach's operation may become too slow.
- Acid works in a similar way – which is why we should not consume too much acid together with high-protein food that is also rich in fat. A small quantity is always desirable, because acid has a favourable effect on the digestion of fat. Fat with acid is a good combination.
- With protein food that is low in fat, on the other hand, we may use more acid because the small quantity of fat has no effect. The acid slows the gastric movement down (acid inhibits acid) so that the high-protein food remains in the stomach longer and is better digested.
- We can mix all kinds of fruit together because they all contain acid and sugar. But it is not possible to tell just by tasting whether a fruit contains a little or a lot of acid. The taste of each fruit is largely the result of its acid-sugar ratio. Do not let the taste mislead you.
- Fruit should be eaten before and not after a meal. Better still: eat fruit separately, as a meal in itself. People who know they are subject to digestive problems should eat only one kind of fruit at a time.
- Maintaining the body's acid-base balance is critical with food combining. If the balance is disturbed, digestion can be problematical even when eating a good combination of foods. We should accordingly always eat small quantities of high-calorie foods in place of large quantities of low-calorie foods. That is a simple but extremely important rule.
- When composing a menu, you should ensure that dishes that follow each other really do go together. The menu must have just a single dominant nutrient, and the acid-base balance must also be taken into consideration.
- The interval between meals is not so important, for the stomach is filled and emptied layer by layer. Whatever we eat first leaves the stomach first; whatever we eat last remains in the stomach the longest. The purpose behind the movements of the gastric wall is to make good contact with the stomach contents so that the gastric juice can fulfil its function, and to press the stomach contents on and down towards the duodenum. The stomach is not a blender that mixes everything together. It should be remembered that the first part of the next meal joins the last part of the previous meal if the stomach has not emptied in between. Because digestion takes place

layer by layer, the stomach does not have to be completely empty in order to eat again.

- All food is bathed in acid in the stomach, and comes into a more alkaline environment in the first part of the duodenum. The small and large intestines form a relatively alkaline chamber in which both fermentation and degradation are possible.
- Vegetables – apart from sauerkraut, those containing lactic acid (such as sweet-sour gherkins pickled in vinegar, or cocktail onions), and tomatoes (if they are vegetables at all) – may be combined with virtually any type of food. Vegetables have a powerfully alkaline effect and are good for the acid-base balance. It is for this reason that we should eat large quantities of vegetables with high-protein foods and foods rich in starch.
- Cooking food makes no difference to food combining. There is no distinction between cooked and raw food. In terms of digestive quality, raw food simply cannot be compared with cooked food – but that is another subject altogether.
- To start food combining, you have only to consult the Diagram of Combinations (p. 99) and follow the guidelines given in this book.
- But it is recommended that any change of dietary regimen should be gradual. Start by eliminating such combinations of foods as protein with starch, and sugar with starch. That represents a great accomplishment in itself. As soon as you are comfortable with that, begin to focus on the positive combinations. Take your time – and avoid nervousness.
- Try also to avoid becoming fanatical about the whole thing. That would be perhaps the worst thing that could befall you. There should be a certain spontaneity about food and about eating, and food combining should likewise have a spontaneous air, comprising dietary rules that are so reasonable that you are glad to keep them, not a rigid system that you feel you must obey come what may. Visiting someone, do not refuse food that constitutes a bad combination: to do so might mean losing friends and other important social contacts. Far better gently to apprise your table-companions of what you do at home, and share with them your enthusiasm for the benefits. Invite your friends to your home and allow them to discover for themselves what food combining might do for them.
- After some months of food combining, you will be more sensitive to combinations of food that are not good ones: you will experience problems if you begin once more to eat as you used to. Then too you will be more aware in life, appreciating that many distracting everyday discomforts in former times were the result of inappropriate combinations of foods.

- Some folk believe food combining to be a method by which to lose weight, a method that should thus not be applied for a long period of time. They are wrong. By food combining, your bodyweight will return to what is normal for it – so fat people will become thinner, and thin people will regain their normal weight. So for people who really are dieting in order to slim it is important, essential even, to follow the principles of food combining.
- When is it best to eat a high-protein meal? That is a question that is frequently put to me. The digestion of protein demands considerable energy, which is why a high-protein breakfast is normally recommended in English-speaking countries. Because the stomach is completely empty and well rested in the morning, that is the time that is generally regarded as best for a high-protein meal. On the other hand, however, people are not exactly wide awake at breakfast-time, and some have very little time anyway for a decent breakfast, so it would seem that there is nothing intrinsically sensible about a high-protein breakfast.

  For many years I have been achieving good results with a light fruit breakfast. It has turned out to be a much better way to start a busy morning. And to tell the truth, there is no genuinely good time to have a large high-protein meal: the intake of high-protein food should always be restricted. So when you eat your high-protein meal does not really matter. It makes no difference whether it is as lunch or as supper. If you do insist on having one, though, it is best to eat it in the evening when, after a day's work, you are relaxed and relaxing.
- The cuisine of other nations around the world is very popular in advanced countries at the moment. All too often, however, it violates the rules of food combining. A Greek salad is a good example of how to eat goat's cheese in a proper way. It is a good combination that works in favour of the acid-base balance. Italian cooking is something else again, dominated by pasta and cheese, a protein-starch combination. It is best to add butter to the pasta: butter as a sauce is less acidic than tomato sauce. Spaghetti and other forms of pasta should be accompanied by vegetables, especially raw vegetables, so that the acid-base balance is maintained. To combine cheese or cheese sauce with spaghetti is horribly wrong.
- Food entering the stomach stimulates the intestines into functioning. Because of this, some people experience a sudden urge to defecate immediately after a meal, and may receive the impression that the food they have just eaten is coming out again. The stimulus relayed by the stomach certainly can increase intestinal peristalsis, which is why we may experience flatulence or intestinal bloating during or after a meal. Because of

the intestinal movement, the intestinal contents start to ferment as the natural process gets under way.

WHEN FOOD COMBINING DOES NOT HELP

It is not impossible that after having followed all these guidelines to the letter, you may still be experiencing wind in the stomach and intestines, you may have neither lost weight nor gained it, you may still be suffering from stomach cramps, and you may not have lost your food allergy. Do not thereupon roundly condemn food combining as an utter waste of time. Something else is likely to be causing your problems. There are ten factors in all that may contribute to digestive problems: they are listed and described below.

1. Disruption of the acid-base balance

No matter how well you practise the principles of food combining, if you do not keep the body's acid-base balance firmly in mind you will go on suffering digestive problems. Two examples.

Bread and cheese is a bad combination. If you add a large quantity of salad or other vegetables, the combination is easier to digest – and that is because the acid-base balance will have been restored.

Meat and vegetables is a good combination. But if you eat a large helping of meat with just a few vegetables, there will be little benefit from the good combination because the acid-base balance will have been disturbed.

Good food combining and the acid-base balance are inextricably linked.

2. Too much food at a time

What is the point of food combining if you stuff your stomach with food anyway? It is very difficult for the stomach to function when it is full to bursting, even if you have been eating food of only the one type. You simply must eat small quantities of food. 'Little and often' is better than one or two huge meals, especially if you are already experiencing digestive problems. The stomach is an organ that more or less works in shifts, processing layer after layer throughout the day, and only emptying completely during the night.

3. Eating too fast

If we eat too fast, we do not chew enough and we swallow lumps that are too big. The purpose behind the stomach's peristalsis is not, as people often imagine, to grind the food but to keep the stomach contents in motion towards the pyloric sphincter and the duodenum. Large lumps of food cannot be completely digested: protein and starch residues are created that may thereafter ferment and degrade in the duodenum and intestines.

4. Swallowing air

It is impossible not to swallow air while eating. But if we eat too fast, we swallow an untoward amount of air, causing us to belch. Air bubbles trapped in the stomach attempt to rise up again into the oesophagus. If gastric acid is present in quantity, some may also be brought up, causing the classic symptoms of acid indigestion.

5. Nervous tension and stress

In many people, the effects of nervous tension are manifested in the stomach and/or the intestines. On occasion the impact is restricted to those organs, but in most cases the entire digestive process is disturbed. These people may well endeavour to practise the principles of food combining, but for them results are pitifully meagre. What they are suffering from is not a nutritional problem but a problem of stress. Eating good combinations of food will improve their digestive processes but will do nothing to cure their troubles. A possible solution in such cases is food combining in association with some carefully chosen relaxation therapy. I have found a form of therapy known as podosegmental reflexology to be an excellent method for dispelling tension in the stomach and intestines, and for gently restoring the nervous system.

6. Disruption of the intestinal flora

The intestinal flora is located at the very end of the small intestine and throughout the large intestine. It comprises a multitude of bacteria which together continue the digestive breakdown of the pulpy chyme, between them digesting the protein and the sugars that remain in the liquid intestinal contents. When there is too much protein or protein residue, those bacteria responsible for breaking down the protein increase rapidly in number at the expense of those bacteria responsible for breaking down the sugars. This is how the intestinal flora is disrupted.

Over time, food combining can beneficially influence the composition of the intestinal flora. But patients suffering from acute intestinal problems need immediate solutions. For as long as their intestinal flora are out of action such people are bound to continue to have intestinal problems. Yoghurt with honey (an acid-sugar combination) can work well by temporarily replacing the flora, as the lactic acid bacteria take over the work of normal intestinal flora. Unfortunately, the effect is shortlived because the lactic acid bacteria are unable to colonize the intestine: they cannot become the intestinal flora. They are a stopgap solution only. The same is true of proprietary preparations based on intestinal bacteria. But yoghurt together with such preparations can help the intestinal flora to function and flourish again.

The intestinal flora may also be attacked and destroyed by certain fungi that may invade the intestine. In such cases, full gastrointestinal examination is essential.

7. Clogged intestines

An intestine that has become befouled and partly clogged through years of eating the wrong things, and especially eating the wrong things together, cannot be cleansed merely by food combining. Food combining will, however, improve the digestion slightly in spite of the disgusting state of the intestine. But such a slight improvement may disillusion some who have made a genuine attempt to try food combining. These people really need to undergo a technique called colonic irrigation, which is a method by which the intestines can be thoroughly cleansed. An apparatus introduces luke-warm water into the large intestine all the way from the rectum back to the ileo-caecal valve at the caecum. Then the water is drained out again while a form of intestinal massage is given. In this way, faecal bits and pieces that may have been stuck on the intestinal wall literally for years are washed off and evacuated through the anus. Patients who apply for this technique should check that their practitioner is qualified to carry it out, and that filtered water is used at all times during the process.

This form of treatment is essential for people who have been following an inappropriate diet for any number of years. Together, a clean intestine and food combining produce very good results.

8. Loss of appetite and eating satisfaction

The nerve centre in the body responsible for sensing appetite and eating satisfaction is the hypothalamus. Seeing, smelling, or even thinking about food stimulates the hypothalamus into action, in turn preparing the digestive system for its own functioning. Such preparation is useful: if we eat when we are not hungry, perhaps because we feel we are too busy to eat, the whole digestion hardly gets moving. We are automatically eating too much because we are not prepared for eating at all. And at the same time we are suffering from stress because of the time factor, unable to think clearly, fearing that we may be falling further behind schedule, and so on. All too frequently, digestive problems are caused by a digestion that is working too slowly because the appetite centre has not been stimulated.

If, on the other hand, it is eating satisfaction that does not register with the hypothalamus, we go on and eat too much. The digestive system then has problems coping with the excessive quantity of food.

Food combining cannot immediately restore a loss of appetite and eating satisfaction because that loss is the result of factors outside its remit (notably stress, tension, emotional problems, or boredom).

9. Gastrointestinal disease

Food combining can provide immediate relief from gastrointestinal disorders, but we should not expect it altogether to cure every problem as quickly. Serious intestinal diseases such as Crohn's disease, a peptic ulcer, or a tumour in the colon cannot be cured by food combining.

10. Eating the wrong types of food together

Bad combinations of food can cause many gastrointestinal disorders, a good few of which may persist so obstinately that a thorough internal examination and a lengthy course of therapy may be required. Food combining always makes sense, and should always be applied, but its results depend on a number of factors. It is not a miracle cure, and we should not expect it to work like one. At the same time it is a fact that many people have been cured of their problems, miraculously or otherwise, by food combining.

Constitutional and other aspects specific to each nonetheless play an important role in our health.

HEALTHY FOOD

There are almost as many ideas about what constitutes healthy food as there are commentators on the subject, some of their ideas contradictory, but all expressed with righteous fervour.

Because food combining is supportive of every diet, I have chosen not to recommend any specific form of dietary regime. The human race has evolved with its own particular digestive system, and I have described it and its function in this book. Whatever eating pattern you adopt, you should take into account what you know of food combining and of the acid-base balance. If you are healthy and do this, you will remain healthy. If you are in poor health, however, it is certainly in your interest to try to improve your diet. Even those whose health is fair can benefit from the extra protection against disease afforded by proper food combining.

This book has already pointed out that a large proportion of the problems to do with diet and health stem from today's exaggerated consumption of agricultural products. To a great extent these products are foisted upon the consuming public because of their economic significance, and are accordingly strongly defended in nutritional reference books. A myth has been created around the eating of meat, cereals and dairy products. We now know, though, that these three foods are problematical in the extreme when combined. They have a seriously disruptive effect on the acid-base balance. If we are really after a healthy diet, we must restrict the eating of agricultural products to a minimum – much less meat, fish, bread, cereals, milk and dairy products. We should eat more, much more, fruit and vegetables. By doing so we will experience fewer problems with food combining and with maintaining the acid-base balance.

Scientific studies have proved that vegetarianism is very healthy, ecologically sound, and morally better in relation to Third World hunger. All nutritionists agree that people in advanced countries eat too much protein. Everyone needs a minimum of 15 grams (½ ounce) of protein per day, on condition that the protein itself is wholesome and contains all the essential amino acids. Because the quality of the protein cannot be guaranteed, 25–30 grams (about an ounce) of protein per person per day should be regarded as the minimum. That is easy to achieve. If the food is combined well, and the acid-base balance is not disturbed, we can count on efficient digestion of the protein. It makes no sense, therefore, to eat as much as 80–100 grams (3–3½ ounces) of protein every day if only a small part of it is put to any real use. In any case, the largest part is damaged and wasted by preparation techniques such as cooking. And if put together in an inappropriate combination of foods, it may remain undigested in the body and degrade there.

Human evolution did not fit us to eat meat or cereals but to eat fruit: we are natural fruit-eaters. Fruit should be regarded as our most basic food. Large amounts of fruit combined correctly or eaten separately offer an inexhaustible source of energy.

We should bear in mind at the same time that tropical and subtropical fruits are comparatively rich and coarse in relation to fruits native to the temperate regions.

I am not trying to coerce you into eating in a new way. I am instead striving to reinforce the point that a healthy diet is more than just food combining. But food combining is a definite step in the right direction.

Food is individual to everyone, and you must decide for yourself, and perhaps for your family, how far you are willing to go. The great value of food combining is that it can be applied by everyone in his or her own eating pattern. To me, that is a tremendous advance.

CONCLUSION

For fifteen years now I have worked as a nutritional therapist. During all these years I have met thousands of people suffering from digestive disorders, many of them seriously ill. I have been able to note in every case just how much of a contributory factor food combining has been to the process of recovery. In addition, it has been a constant pleasure to me to find many doctors now pointing out the benefits of food combining to their patients.

I have considered it my task to investigate food combining on a thorough basis, to judge the combinations critically and to draw conclusions about them, grounding my work on the most up-to-date research into the physiology of digestion. Food combining as I have here presented it is scientifically dependable and dependably scientific. This book is aimed at the widest possible readership, and for that reason I have omitted the studious biological debate and anatomical research that I undertook in the course of putting it together. In a forthcoming textbook for students I will append such further material. Meanwhile, at the back of this book is a full bibliography of reference works I consulted.

As a lecturer in dietetics I am very grateful to my students for the many helpful comments they made during their food combining classes. They have in particular shown and reminded me how much the theories of Dr Hay and Dr Shelton on food combining are no longer up to date and no longer conform to accepted science.

With this book I am hoping to fulfil a great need within the group of people who are searching consciously for the most healthy form of diet. I am also hoping that food combining will at last become part of the overall science of nutrition, for millions of people now experiencing digestive problems can be helped. All they have to do is apply the few simple rules described here. If anyone wants to know more about nutrition and health, he or she may refer to my other published works.

For health and inspiration, my daughter Inge's delicious vegetarian recipes from around the world will show you how to put the theory into practice.

Using these recipes, you will become familiar with the types of food and the combinations of food that are good for you and which will bring relief to your digestive system, and thereby improve your overall health. You will find, in addition, that you are eating food that is delicious and truly good for you at the same time.

Jan Dries

PART II

The Practice

Avocado Stuffed with Raw Vegetables, *see* page 119
Oyster Mushrooms Coated with Breadcrumbs, *see* page 121

Cauliflower–Broccoli Soup, *see* page 131
Pumpkin Soup, *see* page 134
Festive Cream Soup, *see* page 132

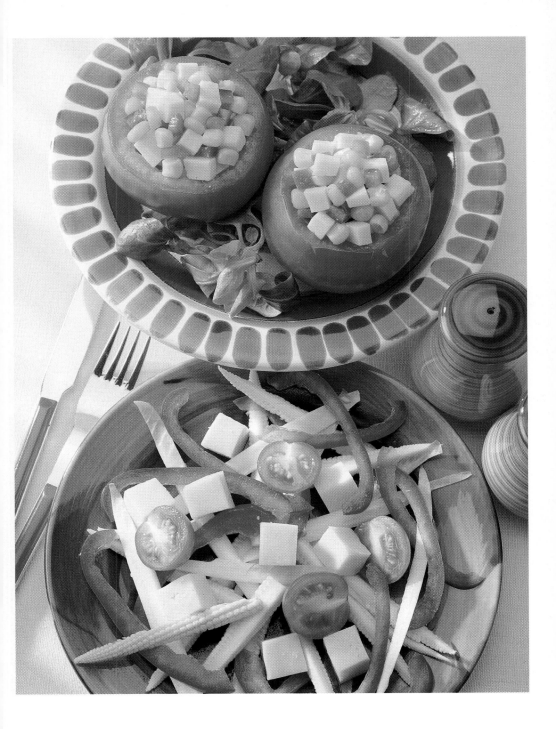

Corn-Cheese Salad, *see* page 139
Mexican Stuffed Tomatoes, *see* page 151

Stuffed Pineapple, *see* page 158
Layers of Fruit Salad, *see* page 162
Fried Banana with Ginger, *see* page 164

BEFORE YOU START . . .

The recipes in this book give quantities in metric and Imperial measures. Remember to follow only one set of measures in a recipe: they are not interchangeable.

These recipes refer to Imperial **pints,** as used in the UK and Australia. An Imperial pint contains 20 fl oz, whereas the US pint is 16 fl oz.

Where quantities are given in **cups**, they refer to the US 8 fl oz measuring cup.

Throughout this book, **tablespoons** refer to the UK standard. This holds 17.7 ml. The US tablespoon holds 14.2 ml and the Australian 20 ml. (A teaspoon is standard at approximately 5 ml.) The table below gives a conversion chart for reference when multiples of tablespoons are required.

British	American	Australian
1 teaspoon	1 teaspoon	1 teaspoon
1 tablespoon	1 tablespoon	1 tablespoon
2 tablespoons	3 tablespoons	2 tablespoons
3½ tablespoons	4 tablespoons	3 tablespoons
4 tablespoons	5 tablespoons	3½ tablespoons

APPETIZERS

STUFFED MUSHROOMS

(serves 4)

20 large mushrooms
1 shallot
1 tbsp butter
1 garlic clove
3 basil leaves
1 parsley sprig
chives
pepper
breadcrumbs
butter
mixed salad

1. Rub the mushrooms clean. (Never wash mushrooms as they absorb water and become spongy.) Remove the stalks and chop finely.
2. Peel the shallot, chop finely and sauté in the butter together with the finely chopped mushroom stalks and garlic.
3. Wash the basil, parsley and chives, pat dry and chop finely. Add the herbs to the mushroom mixture and season with pepper.
4. Fill the mushroom buttons with the mixture and sprinkle with some breadcrumbs.
5. Place some butter on each mushroom and grill until golden brown.
6. Serve on a bed of mixed salad.

(See also recipe on p. 206.)

SOUTHERN TOMATOES

(serves 4)

4 small tomatoes
1 or 2 mozzarella cheeses
4 crinkly lettuce leaves
12 basil leaves

1. Wash the tomatoes, remove the stems and slice.
2. Slice the mozzarella cheese using an egg slicer.
3. Arrange alternate slices of cheese and tomato on top of a lettuce leaf on each of 4 dessert plates.
4. Garnish the salad with basil.

AVOCADO STUFFED WITH RAW VEGETABLES

(serves 4)

2 ripe avocados
1 tbsp lemon juice
4 red lettuce leaves
4 mushrooms
¼ peeled cucumber
4 radishes
1 tbsp oil
½ tbsp lemon juice
fresh herbs

1. Cut the avocados in half, remove the stones and sprinkle the flesh of the fruit with lemon juice to prevent discoloration.
2. Wash the lettuce, pat dry, cut in strips and fill the hollow of the avocado with these strips.
3. Rub the mushrooms clean and slice thinly. Slice the cucumber thinly.
4. Fill the avocado halves with the mushroom and cucumber slices.
5. Garnish with the radishes and pour the dressing consisting of oil, lemon juice and herbs over it.

SPICY MUSHROOM SLICES

(serves 4)

4 slices of bread
herb mayonnaise (see p. 215 for recipe)
4 lettuce leaves
100 g (4 oz) mushrooms
lemon juice
fresh herbs

1. Toast the bread.
2. Spread the toast with the herb mayonnaise.
3. Wash the lettuce, pat dry, cut into strips and place on the toast.
4. Rub the mushrooms clean, slice thinly and arrange on top of the lettuce.
5. Sprinkle with lemon juice and garnish with fresh, finely chopped herbs.

SCRAMBLED EGGS WITH FRESH HERBS

(serves 4)

4 brown eggs
2 tbsp fresh chopped herbs
1 tbsp oil
chives

1. Take the eggs and carefully crack the shell at the smaller end. (The shells are needed later in the recipe.) Pour the contents of the eggs into a bowl and whisk until frothy.
2. Blend the herbs with the eggs.
3. Heat the oil, add the eggs and allow to set while stirring constantly.
4. Carefully rinse the eggshells with water and fill them with the scrambled eggs. Place the eggs in 4 attractive egg-cups (preferably with a high base) and garnish with a few blades of chives.

GARLIC TOMATOES

(serves 4)

1 small bowl cherry tomatoes
a few leaves of lettuce
3 parsley sprigs
3 basil leaves
1 garlic clove
1 tbsp oil

1. Wash the tomatoes, dry and remove the stems.
2. Wash the parsley and basil, dry and chop finely. Peel the garlic and chop finely.
3. Heat the oil and sauté the tomatoes, sprinkling the garlic and herbs onto them.
4. Serve the tomatoes on a bed of lettuce.

STUFFED ARTICHOKE

(serves 4)

4 medium-sized globe artichokes
3 tbsp mayonnaise
1 tbsp yoghurt
2 tbsp fresh herbs, chopped
2 pickled gherkins
1 shallot
pepper
paprika
salt

1. Thoroughly wash the artichokes, cut the stalks and cook in a saucepan of water. An artichoke is ready when its base can be pierced with a fork. Take the artichokes out of the water and let them cool.
2. Remove the middle part (the small leaves) from the artichokes, making the heart visible. Remove the hearts and cut off pieces at the bottom, so that the artichokes will stand up.
3. Blend the mayonnaise, yoghurt and herbs.
4. Finely chop the gherkins. Peel the shallot and slice thinly. Blend both into the sauce.
5. Season the sauce with pepper, paprika and salt.
6. Fill the hollow of the artichokes with the sauce and serve. Peel off the leaves of the artichoke one by one and dip them in the sauce. The lower part of each leaf is edible, the rest is not. After you have eaten the leaves and finished the sauce, you will find the delicious base.

OYSTER MUSHROOMS COATED WITH BREADCRUMBS

(serves 4)

400 g (14 oz) small oyster mushrooms
1 egg white
3 or 4 tbsp breadcrumbs and/or sesame seeds
oil or butter

1. Wipe the mushrooms (do not wash).
2. Beat the egg white and pour into a soup plate.
3. Put the breadcrumbs or sesame seeds onto 1 or 2 plates.
4. First, dip the mushrooms in the egg white, then in the breadcrumbs and/or the sesame seeds.
5. Fry the mushrooms in the oil or butter until they are golden brown.

FENNEL AU GRATIN

(serves 4)

2 fennel roots
pepper
paprika
4 slices Camembert cheese
curly endive

1. Cut the fennel roots in half, wash and cook or steam.
2. Put the halved fennel roots in a greased, heat-resistant oven dish and sprinkle with pepper and paprika.
3. Place the Camembert over the fennel and grill.
4. Serve on 4 plates, garnished with the endive.

AVOCADO DIP

(serves 4)

2 avocados
1 tbsp lemon juice
4 radishes
3 basil leaves
lettuce
tacos

1. Cut the avocados in half, remove the stones and scoop out the flesh with a teaspoon. (The shells will be needed later in the recipe.)
2. Purée the flesh in a blender until smooth. Add lemon juice to prevent discoloration.
3. Wash the radishes, dry and slice thinly.
4. Fill the hollow shells with the avocado purée and garnish with the radish slices.
5. Wash the basil, pat dry, shred finely and sprinkle onto the avocados.
6. Serve the avocados halves on 4 small plates with lettuce and warm tacos.

TASTY CROISSANTS

(serves 4)

3 or 4 (frozen) squares of puff pastry

6 mushrooms

garlic

pepper

fresh herbs

2 sautéed shallots

3 tbsp fried vegetables (onions, carrots, broccoli, etc.)

1. Defrost the pastry 15 minutes before it is needed.
2. Cut each square diagonally to form 4 triangles.
3. Rub the mushrooms clean, slice and sauté adding a little garlic and pepper.
4. Fill ⅓ of the triangles with the mushroom mixture and roll into croissants. Fill ½ of the remaining pastry with fresh herbs and sautéed shallot.
5. Fill the rest of the pastry with fried vegetables.
6. Bake the croissants in a preheated oven for 10 to 15 minutes.

EASTER EGG NESTS

(serves 4)

½ head of lettuce

3 eggs

12 cherry tomatoes

herb mayonnaise (see p. 215 for recipe)

1. Wash the lettuce, dry and cut into strips. Form a 'nest' of lettuce on 4 plates.
2. Hard boil the eggs. Let them cool and cut lengthwise into 4 slices. Fill each nest with 3 slices of egg.
3. Wash the tomatoes, dry and divide among the nests.
4. Serve with herb mayonnaise.

STUFFED EGGS

(serves 4)

a few lettuce leaves

4 eggs

1 or 2 tbsp mayonnaise

1 tsp curry powder

mustard and cress

1. Wash the lettuce, dry and spread over 4 plates.
2. Hard boil the eggs. Let them cool and cut in half. Remove the egg yolks, mash and blend with the mayonnaise and curry powder.
3. Use a piping bag to fill the eggs with the yolk mixture. Arrange the stuffed eggs on the plates and garnish with mustard and cress.

SOUPS

VEGETABLE STOCK

3 litres (7 pints; 16 cups) water
1 celeriac
2 onions
1 carrot
2 leeks
pepper
1 tbsp salt
2 garlic cloves
2 bay leaves

For a quick stock use instant vegetable stock granules or bouillon powder, which can also be used for seasoning instead of salt. For homemade vegetable stock:

1. Clean the vegetables and cut into pieces.
2. Put the vegetables into a large pan of hot water with the pepper, salt, garlic and bay leaves.
3. Simmer with the lid on for 2 hours.
4. Strain the stock through a sieve and use as required. (The stock can be frozen and used later.)

CLEAR VEGETABLE SOUP OR CONSOMMÉ

(serves 4)

1 large carrot
½ small celeriac
1 red pepper
1 small courgette (zuccini)
1 shallot
1 tbsp oil
1 litre (1¾ pints; 4 cups) vegetable stock (see above for recipe)
parsley

1. Wash or peel the carrot and slice.
2. Peel the celeriac and cut into strips.
3. Wash the red pepper, remove the seeds and cut into strips.
4. Wash the courgette and use a small melon scoop to remove the seeds.
5. Thinly slice the shallot.
6. Heat the oil and sauté the shallot. Add the sliced vegetables and cook gently for a while. Add the stock and bring to the boil, making sure the soup does not boil for more than 2 minutes.
7. Serve with finely chopped parsley.

RAW VEGETABLE SOUP

(serves 4)

1 carrot
½ shallot
½ small celeriac
¼ cucumber
1 litre (1¾ pints; 4 cups) vegetable
  stock (see p. 126 for recipe)
parsley

1. Wash or peel the carrot.
2. Peel the shallot, celeriac and cucumber and cut into pieces.
3. Put the vegetables in a blender with the hot stock.
4. Garnish with finely chopped parsley. Serve hot or cold.

CREAMY CUCUMBER SOUP WITH DILL

(serves 4)

1 large cucumber
1 tbsp butter
2 tbsp flour
1 litre (1¾ pints; 4 cups) vegetable
  stock (see p. 126 for recipe)
3 dill sprigs
cream

1. Peel the cucumber, cut into pieces and purée in a blender (add water if necessary).
2. Heat the butter in a pan and stir in the flour (creating a roux).
3. When the butter has absorbed the flour completely, add the stock stirring constantly. Add the cucumber purée and let the soup heat through until creamy, stirring occasionally.
4. Wash the dill, pat dry, chop finely and add just before serving. For a special occasion, add a splash of cream to the soup.

(This recipe can be used for converting all vegetables into a creamy soup.)

GAZPACHO

(serves 4)

1 cucumber
1 red pepper
3 large beefsteak tomatoes
1 shallot
½ tbsp olive oil
2 garlic cloves
parsley

1. Peel the cucumber.
2. Wash the red pepper and remove the seeds.
3. Skin the tomatoes and remove the seeds.
4. Peel the shallot.
5. Cut all the vegetables into pieces and put in a blender with the oil and garlic.
6. Serve cold and garnish with finely chopped pepper, cucumber and parsley if required.

LEEK SOUP

(serves 4)

3 leeks
1 tbsp butter or margarine
1 tbsp flour
1 litre (1¾ pints; 4 cups) vegetable stock (see p. 126 for recipe)
pepper
1 tbsp fresh lemon balm, chopped

1. Remove the dark green part from the leeks. Wash the rest thoroughly and slice into rings. Stew the leek in butter or margarine.
2. Heat the butter or margarine and stir in the flour.
3. When the butter has absorbed the flour completely, add the stock, stirring constantly. Add the leek and let the soup heat through for a few minutes.
4. Season the soup with pepper. Just before serving, add the lemon balm.

For a special occasion, stir in some cream.

ONION SOUP

(serves 4)

4 large onions
2 potatoes
1 tbsp butter
1 litre (1¾ pints; 4 cups) vegetable
   stock (see p. 126 for recipe)
2 bay leaves
chives
croûtons

1. Peel and finely chop the onions.
2. Peel the potatoes and cut into cubes.
3. Heat the butter and sauté the onions and the potatoes.
4. Add the stock and bay leaves.
5. Let the soup cook for 10 minutes, then blend if preferred.
6. Garnish with chives and croûtons if required.

RAW TOMATO SOUP

(serves 4)

3 tomatoes
½ cucumber
½ shallot
1 stick celery
1 litre (1¾ pints; 4 cups) vegetable
   stock (see p. 126 for recipe)
fresh basil, chopped

1. Skin the tomatoes and remove the seeds.
2. Peel the cucumber and shallots, chop finely and put in a blender with the tomatoes.
3. Wash the celery, chop finely and blend with the other vegetables.
4. Meanwhile, boil the stock. Mix the vegetables with the hot stock and season with basil.
5. Serve the soup immediately.

MUSHROOM SOUP

(serves 4)

250 g (9 oz) mushrooms
1 tbsp butter
1 tbsp flour
1 litre (1¾ pints; 4 cups) vegetable stock (see p. 126 for recipe)
pepper
fresh parsley, chopped

1. Rub the mushrooms clean, slice and sauté in the butter.
2. Add the flour, while stirring constantly.
3. When the butter has absorbed the flour completely, add the stock.
4. Add the mushrooms and let the soup cook for a few minutes. Season the soup with pepper.
5. Garnish with parsley.

(This recipe can be used for turning all vegetables into a creamy soup.)

CLEAR BOUILLON SOUP

(serves 4)

1 carrot
100 g (4 oz) mushrooms
6 small cauliflower florets
1 leek
1 tbsp oil
1 litre (1¾ pints; 4 cups) vegetable stock (see p. 126 for recipe)
1 tbsp soy sauce
pepper
lettuce leaves

1. Peel the carrot and cut into even slices of more or less 1 mm width.
2. Rub the mushrooms clean, remove the lower part of the stalks and slice.
3. Wash the cauliflower.
4. Wash the leek, remove any roots and green parts and slice into rings.
5. Heat the oil and sauté the vegetables in it for a short time only.
6. Add the stock and let the soup cook for no longer than 2 minutes in order to keep the vegetables crisp. Season with soy sauce.
7. Just before serving, arrange 2 lettuce leaves on each plate. Pour the broth over the lettuce and serve hot.

CAULIFLOWER-BROCCOLI SOUP

(serves 4)

½ small cauliflower
1 small broccoli head
1 shallot
1 carrot
1 tbsp oil
1 litre (1¾ pints; 4 cups) vegetable stock (see p. 126 for recipe)
pepper
fresh herbs, chopped

1. Thoroughly wash the cauliflower and separate into florets.
2. Do the same with the broccoli.
3. Peel the shallot and carrot and cut finely.
4. Gently cook the vegetables in the oil for 2 minutes. Add the stock and let the soup simmer for 2 or 3 minutes only, so that the cauliflower and the broccoli remain crisp.
5. Season with pepper and garnish with fresh herbs.

CREAMY ASPARAGUS SOUP

(serves 4)

1 bundle of asparagus
1 litre (1¾ pints; 4 cups) vegetable stock (see p. 126 for recipe)
1 tbsp butter
1 tbsp flour
3 tbsp cream
fresh dill

1. Wash the asparagus, removing the fibrous lower part (but save it for the stock, together with the skins) and cut the asparagus into equal pieces.
2. Prepare a vegetable stock and add the asparagus skins and fibrous parts. Heat the butter and stir the flour into it.
3. When the butter has absorbed the flour completely, add the strained stock and asparagus pieces, but set aside the asparagus tips. Let the soup cook until the asparagus pieces are well done. Five minutes before serving the soup, add the asparagus tips.
4. When the soup is ready, add the cream and garnish with dill.

FESTIVE CREAM SOUP

(serves 4)

1 leek
1 fennel root
1 celery stalk
1 shallot
1 carrot
1 tbsp butter
1 litre (1¾ pints; 4 cups) vegetable stock (see p. 126 for recipe)
saffron
3 thyme sprigs
125 ml (¼ pint; ½ cup) cream

1. Clean (removing any roots and green parts), wash and shred the leek and fennel root.
2. Peel and shred the celery, shallot and carrot.
3. Heat the butter and cook the vegetables for a short time only.
4. Add the stock, saffron and thyme.
5. Bring the soup to the boil and let it cook for 5 to 10 minutes.
6. Just before serving, add the cream.

CELERIAC SOUP

(serves 4)

1 celeriac
1 large potato
2 carrots
1 onion
1 tbsp oil
1.5 litre (2½ pints; 6 cups) vegetable stock (see p. 126 for recipe)
1 bay leaf
parsley

1. Peel and cut the celeriac, potato, carrots and onion into cubes.
2. Heat the oil and sauté the vegetables for a short time only.
3. Add the stock and let the soup cook until the vegetables are ready.
4. Put the soup in a blender and when smooth sprinkle with some parsley.

AVOCADO SOUP

(serves 4)

2 avocados
1 litre (1¾ pints; 4 cups) vegetable
stock (see p. 126 for recipe)
pepper
fresh herbs

1. Peel the avocados, remove the stones and cut the flesh into pieces.
2. Meanwhile, boil the stock.
3. Add the avocado to the stock and transfer to a blender.
4. Season with pepper and garnish with fresh herbs.

CHINESE VEGETABLE SOUP

(serves 4)

2 spring onions
½ red pepper
150 g (5 oz) beansprouts
1 carrot
1 tbsp oil
1 tbsp soy sauce
1 litre (1¾ pints; 4 cups) cold
vegetable stock (see p. 126
for recipe)
5 lettuce leaves
pepper

1. Clean the spring onions, removing the roots and any withered green parts. Slice them, finely cut the green parts and use them to garnish the soup.
2. Wash the red pepper, remove the seeds and cut into thin strips.
3. Wash the beansprouts and remove the dark roots.
4. Peel the carrot and slice thinly.
5. Heat the oil and sauté the vegetables for a short time only.
6. Add the soy sauce and the stock and bring to the boil.
7. Just before serving, add the lettuce to the soup and garnish with the onion greens. Season with pepper.

PUMPKIN SOUP

(serves 4)

1 small pumpkin
1 onion
1 tbsp oil
1.5 litres (2½ pints; 6 cups)
vegetable stock (see p. 126
for recipe)
fresh parsley, chopped

1. Peel the pumpkin and cut into pieces, discarding the seeds.
2. Peel and slice the onion.
3. Heat the oil and sauté the pumpkin and onion.
4. Add the stock and cook the soup until the vegetables are ready.
5. Put the soup in a blender and garnish with parsley.

MINESTRONE

(serves 4)

1 carrot
1 celery stalk
¼ cauliflower
1 large potato
¼ celeriac
1 tbsp oil
1.5 litres (2½ pints; 6 cups)
vegetable stock (see p. 126
for recipe)
1 tsp basil
1 tsp oregano
pepper
Parmesan cheese

1. Peel the carrot and cut into strips.
2. Wash the celery stalk and cut into pieces.
3. Wash the cauliflower and separate into florets.
4. Peel the potato and cut into cubes.
5. Heat the oil and sauté the vegetables for a short time only.
6. Add the stock and cook the soup for 10 minutes.
7. Season with basil, oregano and freshly ground pepper. To add an Italian touch, sprinkle with some grated Parmesan cheese.

FINE HERB CREAM SOUP

(serves 4)

2 tbsp mixed, fresh, herbs minced, (e.g. tarragon, fennel, chervil, chives, basil)

½ onion

½ leek

1 fennel root

1 celery stalk

1 tbsp butter

1.5 litres (2½ pints; 6 cups) vegetable stock (see p. 126 for recipe)

cream

basil

1. Peel the onion and chop finely.
2. Clean the leek (removing any roots and green parts), fennel root and celery, and finely chop.
3. Heat the butter in a large saucepan, add the vegetables and sauté for a while.
4. Add the stock and bring the soup to the boil. Add the herbs and blend the soup if required.
5. Just before serving, stir in some cream. Decorate the soup with a few leaves of basil.

COLD CUCUMBER SOUP

(serves 4)

1 cucumber

½ litre (1 pint; 2 cups) yoghurt

½ lemon

3 fresh mint leaves

½ tbsp chives, chopped

1 garlic clove, minced

1 parsley sprig, chopped

1. Peel the cucumber and shred or purée.
2. Add the yoghurt and the juice of half a lemon.
3. Season with mint, chives, garlic and parsley.

(This is very refreshing in hot weather.)

ARTICHOKE BISQUE

(serves 4)

3 large globe artichokes
1 tbsp lemon juice
2 tbsp olive oil
2 garlic cloves, minced
1 litre (1¾ pints; 4 cups) water
1 small onion
1 tbsp butter
700 ml (1¼ pints; 3 cups)
  vegetable stock (see p. 126
  for recipe)
cayenne pepper
fresh basil
125 ml (¼ pint; ½ cup) cream

1. Wash the artichokes and cut off the stalks, leaving 1 cm (½ inch). Bend the outermost leaves until they break off and then cut the rest of the leaves off, leaving the lower part. Separate the leaves from the bases.

2. Bring the lemon juice, olive oil, water and garlic to the boil, and cook the artichoke bases in this. The bases are ready when they can be easily pierced with a fork.

3. Set aside 375 ml (¾ pint; 1½ cups) of the cooking water. Gently boil the leaves. After 20 minutes, drain the leaves and use a spoon to remove and separate the edible pulp. Remove the heart from the artichoke bases and cut off the remaining leaves at the edges.

4. Peel the onion, shred and sauté in the butter.

5. Add the artichoke liquid and stock to the onion.

6. Add the pulp and the chopped artichoke bases to the soup. Let the soup heat through for a while and purée.

7. Season with cayenne pepper and basil. Add the cream and serve the soup hot.

SALADS

GARDENER'S SALAD

(serves 4)

½ head of lettuce
½ cauliflower
200 g (7 oz) French beans
2 tomatoes
½ cucumber
fresh parsley, chopped
salad dressing or mayonnaise
(see *Dressings and Sauces* for recipes)

1. Wash and dry the lettuce.
2. Wash and separate the cauliflower into florets.
3. Steam or boil the cauliflower and allow to cool.
4. Clean the French beans. Steam or cook and let them cool.
5. Wash the tomatoes and cut into pieces.
6. Peel the cucumber and slice thinly.
7. Arrange the vegetables on a large dish and sprinkle with the parsley.
8. Serve the salad with a salad dressing or with mayonnaise.

FINE ASPARAGUS SALAD

(serves 4)

1 bundle green asparagus
1 bundle white asparagus
mustard sauce (see p. 216 for recipe)
mustard and cress

1. Carefully peel the green and white asparagus.
2. Remove the fibrous parts and cut the asparagus into equal pieces. Set aside the asparagus tips. Cook the rest in water. Do not add the asparagus tips until the last 5 minutes.
3. Drain the asparagus on an asparagus dish or on a clean table napkin.
4. Put the asparagus on a dish and coat with mustard sauce. Garnish with mustard and cress.

CORN-CHEESE SALAD

(serves 4)

150 g (5 oz) cooked sweetcorn or minicobs

150 g (5 oz) gouda cheese

6 endive leaves

½ red pepper

8 cherry tomatoes

salad dressing or mayonnaise (see *Dressings and Sauces* for recipes)

1. Remove the rind from the cheese and cut into cubes and add to the drained corn.
2. Wash the endive leaves and cut into strips.
3. Wash the red pepper, remove the seeds and slice thinly.
4. Wash and cut the tomatoes in half.
5. Add all vegetables to the cheese and corn and toss the salad until well mixed.
6. Serve with a salad dressing or with mayonnaise.

POTATO SALAD

(serves 4)

600 g (1 lb 4 oz) potatoes

2 shallots

5 tbsp mayonnaise (see p. 214 for recipe)

chives

parsley

1. Thoroughly scrub the potatoes and boil them in their skins. Let them cool, peel and slice them.
2. Peel the shallots, chop finely and add to the potato slices.
3. Add the mayonnaise.
4. Wash, pat dry and finely chop the chives and parsley and blend with the potato salad.

(See also recipe on p. 187.)

AVOCADO WITH LAMB'S LETTUCE

(serves 2)

300 g (11 oz) lamb's lettuce
2 ripe avocados
lemon juice
pepper
basil
12 cherry tomatoes
1 yellow pepper

1. Wash the lettuce, dry and divide among 4 plates.
2. Peel the avocados and remove the stones. Slice 1 avocado and sprinkle with lemon juice to avoid discoloration. Arrange the avocado slices on the 4 plates.
3. Purée the other avocado, add lemon juice, and flavour with pepper and basil.
4. Divide the purée among the plates and garnish with the tomatoes and cubes of yellow pepper.

STUFFED TOMATOES FROM WARMER REGIONS

(serves 2)

4 large beefsteak tomatoes
¼ courgette (zuccini)
¼ yellow pepper
2 tbsp boiled sweetcorn
5 green pitted olives
1 fresh tarragon sprig
2 tbsp vinaigrette (see p. 214 for recipe)
½ tsp mustard
curly endive

1. Wash the tomatoes, dry, cut off the bottom and carefully scoop out with a teaspoon. Put the tomatoes upside down on a plate, allowing the juice to drain. Set aside the tomato flesh for preparing a soup.
2. Peel and shred the courgette.
3. Wash the pepper, remove the seeds, shred and blend with the courgette.
4. Add the sweetcorn, together with the olives, cut into pieces, and the tarragon.
5. Pour the vinaigrette and mustard onto the salad and refrigerate for an hour.
6. Fill the tomatoes with the salad and garnish them with a few leaves of endive.

FESTIVE RED CHICORY SALAD

(serves 2)

3 red chicory spears
100 g (4 oz) lamb's lettuce
100 g (4 oz) curly endive
6 radishes
2 tbsp walnut oil
½ tbsp ground mustard seeds
1½ tbsp lemon juice
cayenne pepper
10 shelled walnuts

1. Wash the chicory, remove the bitter core and chop finely.
2. Wash the lettuce and endive, pat dry (finely cut the curly endive) and add to the red chicory.
3. Wash the radishes, remove any green parts, slice and blend with the salad.
4. Blend the walnut oil, mustard seeds and lemon juice and season with cayenne pepper.
5. Garnish with the walnuts.

RED CABBAGE SALAD

(serves 2)

¼ small red cabbage
1 shallot
1½ tbsp red wine vinegar
1 tsp mustard
4 tbsp olive oil
parsley

1. Wash the red cabbage, dry and slice finely (using bread-slicer or food processor).
2. Peel the shallot, slice and add the vinegar, mustard and olive oil.
3. Pour the dressing onto the red cabbage and garnish with parsley.
4. Refrigerate the red cabbage salad for a few hours (preferably overnight) before serving.

MIXED SALAD WITH ROASTED SESAME SEEDS

(serves 2)

400 g (14 oz) mixed greens
(e.g. crinkly lettuce, endive
salad, raddichio, lamb's lettuce)
2 tbsp walnut oil
3 tbsp sesame seeds

1. Wash the mixed greens, dry and tear into small pieces.
2. Put the salad in a large bowl and coat with walnut oil.
3. Lightly roast the sesame seeds in a pan and sprinkle on to the salad.

(You can also use pine nuts, croûtons, sunflower seeds, etc.)

GREEK SALAD

(serves 2)

150 g (5 oz) lamb's lettuce
½ raddichio
4 curly endive leaves
150 g (5 oz) Feta cheese
5 black olives
5 green olives
1 green pepper
3 or 4 tbsp vinaigrette (see p. 214 for recipe)

1. Wash the lettuce, dry and put on to a dish.
2. Wash the raddichio and endive, cut in strips and add to the lettuce.
3. Cut the Feta cheese into cubes and spread over the salad.
4. Garnish with the black and green olives and green pepper.
5. Coat with vinaigrette and serve.

142

SOUTHERN POTATO SALAD

(serves 2)

500 g (1 lb 2 oz) potatoes
½ head of lettuce
6 green stuffed olives
2 tbsp olive oil
1 tsp mustard
fresh oregano

1. Scrub the potatoes and boil in their skins. Allow them to cool and then slice them.
2. Wash the lettuce, dry, arrange on a dish and put the potatoes on top.
3. Garnish the salad with green olives, sliced thinly.
4. Prepare a dressing of olive oil, mustard and fresh oregano. Pour this dressing on to the potatoes and serve.

ASPARAGUS–AVOCADO SALAD

(serves 4)

500 g (1 lb 2 oz) mixed
  asparagus (white and green)
4 lettuce leaves
100 g (5 oz) mushrooms
1 avocado
1½ tbsp sherry vinegar
3 tbsp oil
1 tbsp mustard seed, ground
mustard and cress

1. Carefully peel the asparagus and cut into equal pieces. Cook the asparagus pieces (do not add the tips until the last 5 minutes). Allow the asparagus to cool and then drain. Put the pieces on a dish.
2. Wash the lettuce, pat dry and tear into small pieces.
3. Rub the mushrooms clean and slice thinly. Blend the lettuce with the asparagus and the mushrooms.
4. Peel the avocado, remove the stone, cut into cubes and sprinkle with lemon juice to avoid discoloration.
5. Mix the avocado cubes with the salad and coat with a dressing made from sherry vinegar, oil and ground mustard seed.
6. Garnish the salad with mustard and cress.

SOUTHERN RED CHICORY SALAD

(serves 2)

1 yellow pepper
2 spears red chicory
5 green stuffed olives
2 tomatoes
2 tbsp mustard
3 tbsp olive oil
fresh basil
paprika
pepper

1. Wash the yellow pepper, remove the seeds and cut into pieces.
2. Wash the red chicory, pat dry, slice thinly and blend with the pepper.
3. Slice the green olives.
4. Wash the tomatoes, slice and mix with the salad together with the olives. Coat with a dressing made from mustard and olive oil.
5. Season with fresh basil, pepper and paprika.

NEW ORLEANS COLESLAW

(serves 4)

¼ red cabbage
¼ white cabbage
3 carrots
3 spring onions
½ yellow pepper
60 ml (⅛ pint; ¼ cup) sour cream
60 ml (⅛ pint; ¼ cup) mayonnaise
  (see p. 214 for recipe)
2 tbsp lemon juice
1 tbsp fresh parsley, chopped
1 tbsp celery leaf, chopped
1 tbsp onion, shredded
cayenne pepper

1. Wash the red and white cabbages, cut into strips (using a bread-slicer or a shredder).
2. Peel and shred the carrots.
3. Wash the spring onions, remove the roots and slice finely.
4. Wash the yellow pepper, remove the seeds and cut into strips. Put the vegetables in a bowl and mix.
5. Blend the sour cream, mayonnaise and lemon juice. Season this dressing with fresh parsley, celery leaf, shredded onion and cayenne pepper. Thoroughly blend the dressing with the vegetables.

RADICCHIO SALAD

(serves 4)

1 radicchio	1. Wash the radicchio and cut finely.
100 g (4 oz) lamb's lettuce	2. Wash the lettuce, pat dry and add to the
1 avocado	radicchio.
lemon juice	3. Peel the avocado, remove the stone and cut
1 tsp mustard	the flesh into pieces. Sprinkle the avocado with
3 tbsp yoghurt	lemon juice (to avoid discoloration) and blend
1 tbsp mayonnaise (see p. 214	with the salad.
for recipe)	4. Prepare a dressing of mustard, yoghurt and
pepper	mayonnaise. Season with pepper. Garnish with
fresh herbs	some chopped herbs.

CREAMY CUCUMBER SALAD

(serves 2)

1 cucumber	1. Peel the cucumber and slice thinly (in a
½ shallot	food processor).
125 ml (¼ pint; ½ cup) cream	2. Peel the shallot, chop finely and add to the
1 tbsp mayonnaise (see p. 214	cucumber.
for recipe)	3. Add the cream and mayonnaise. Season with
1 tbsp parsley, chopped	parsley, dill and if necessary, salt.
1 tbsp dill, chopped	
salt	

TOMATOES WITH CURD CHEESE FILLING

(serves 2)

4 tomatoes
200 g (7 oz) low-fat curd cheese
100 g (4 oz) (unsweetened)
  whipped cream
pepper
10 leaves of basil

1. Wash and dry the tomatoes. Cut off the bottom part and scoop out the flesh using a teaspoon. Drain the tomatoes upside down on a plate.
2. Blend low-fat curd cheese with the cream and pepper.
3. Wash the basil, pat dry and chop finely.
4. Blend the basil with the mixture and fill the tomatoes with this mixture. Serve on a bed of lettuce.

WHITE CABBAGE SALAD

(serves 4)

600 g (1 lb 5 oz) white cabbage
1 garlic clove, minced
1 tbsp white wine vinegar
4 tbsp water
pepper
oregano
salt

1. Wash the white cabbage and cut into strips (using a bread-slicer or food processor). Boil the cabbage strips for 5 minutes and strain.
2. Meanwhile, prepare a dressing of garlic, vinegar, water, pepper, oregano and, if necessary, salt.
3. Pour the dressing on to the hot cabbage strips and allow it to marinate for a few hours.

CELERIAC SALAD

(serves 4)

1 celeriac
1 lemon
2 tbsp mayonnaise (see p. 214 for recipe)
fresh chives

1. Peel and shred the celeriac. Add the lemon juice to avoid discoloration.
2. Add the mayonnaise and blend with the celeriac.
3. Wash the chives and shred over the salad.

(This salad can also be prepared with carrots or a combination of carrots and celeriac.)

WHITE CABBAGE DRESSED FOR SUMMER

(serves 4)

¼ white cabbage
1 cup vinaigrette (see p. 214 for recipe)
200 g (7 oz) lamb's lettuce
black olives
½ red pepper
½ green pepper
tomato slices
cucumber

1. Wash the white cabbage, dry, shred and add the vinaigrette. Toss and set aside for a couple of hours.
2. Wash the lettuce, dry and arrange on a dish.
3. Put the cabbage on top of the lettuce and garnish with black olives, peppers, tomato slices and cucumber.

CORN SALAD

(serves 4)

250 g (9 oz) cooked sweetcorn	1. Drain the sweetcorn.
2 young carrots	2. Peel the carrots and courgette and slice thinly.
1 small courgette (zuccini)	3. Wash and cut the tomatoes in half.
12 cherry tomatoes	4. Wash the green pepper, remove the seeds and cut into strips.
1 green pepper	
½ red onion	5. Peel the onion and slice into thin rings.
100 g (3 oz) black olives	6. Put all the vegetables into a large bowl with the black olives and the capers and mix well.
2 tsp capers	
6 tbsp olive oil	7. Make the dressing by blending the olive oil, vinegar, lime juice, mustard and fresh tarragon. Season with cayenne pepper.
3 tbsp white wine vinegar	
1 tsp lime juice	
1 tsp mustard	
1 tbsp fresh tarragon, minced	
cayenne pepper	

SOUTHERN SALAD

(serves 2)

½ cucumber	1. Peel and slice the cucumber.
2 tomatoes	2. Wash the tomatoes, slice and add to the cucumber slices.
½ onion	
½ yellow pepper	3. Peel the onions and cut into rings.
½ red pepper	4. Wash the yellow and red peppers, remove the seeds and cut into strips. Mix with the cucumber, tomato and onion.
125 ml (¼ pint; ½ cup) vinaigrette (see p. 214 for recipe)	
6 black olives	5. Coat with the vinaigrette and set aside in the refrigerator for an hour.
	6. Garnish with black olives.

LEEK SALAD

(serves 4)

8 leeks
1 garlic clove
1 tsp mustard
125 ml (¼ pint; ½ cup) oil
60 ml (⅛ pint; ¼ cup) white wine
  vinegar
1 tbsp fresh lemon juice
chives, chopped

1. Wash the leeks (removing any roots and green parts) and boil for 15 minutes with the garlic. Drain the leeks and arrange on a dish.
2. Blend the mustard, oil, vinegar and lemon juice and pour on to the leeks.
3. Garnish with chives. Put the leek salad in the refrigerator for 1 or 2 hours, allowing the dressing to soak in.

SPICY OYSTER MUSHROOM SALAD

(serves 4)

300 g (11 oz) oyster mushrooms
1 tbsp butter
1 garlic clove
chicken spices (a spicy mixture of
  herbs for chicken dishes)
cayenne pepper
1 head of lettuce
10 cherry tomatoes
50 g (2 oz) pecan nuts
½ tsp fresh thyme

1. Rub the mushrooms clean and fry in butter with the garlic.
2. Sprinkle the mushrooms with the chicken spices and cayenne pepper. Cook until brown.
3. Wash the lettuce, dry and tear. Put it in a bowl and mix with the mushrooms, tomatoes, pecan nuts and thyme.

SPICY AVOCADO

(appetizer for 2)

1 ripe avocado
1 green celery stalk
1 tbsp lemon juice
1 tsp curry powder
4 red lettuce leaves
2 slices lemon
2 black olives

1. Cut the avocado in half and remove the stone. Carefully scoop out the flesh and purée with the washed celery. Add lemon juice to prevent discoloration and flavour with curry powder.
2. Wash the lettuce, pat dry and arrange on 2 plates. Fill the avocado halves with the avocado purée.
3. Garnish with lemon slices and black olives.

MUSHROOM SALAD

(side dish for 4)

250 g (9 oz) mushrooms
lemon juice
½ onion
1 bundle chervil
chives
125 ml (¼ pint; ½ cup) vinaigrette
  (see p. 214 for recipe)
1 garlic clove, minced

1. Rub the mushrooms clean and remove the lower parts of the stalks. Slice the mushrooms and sprinkle with lemon juice.
2. Peel and finely chop the onion.
3. Wash and chop the chervil and a few blades of chives. Mix with the mushrooms and the finely chopped onion.
4. Season with garlic. Pour on to the mushroom salad. Refrigerate for an hour.

MIXED SALAD WITH TOMATO VINAIGRETTE

(serves 2)

½ cucumber

2 tomatoes

½ yellow pepper

3 leaves Chinese cabbage or iceberg lettuce

tomato vinaigrette (see p. 214 for recipe)

1. Peel and slice the cucumber.
2. Wash the tomatoes, cut into pieces and add to the cucumber.
3. Wash the yellow pepper, remove the seeds and cut finely.
4. Wash the cabbage or lettuce and cut into strips. Mix the vegetables well and serve with a tomato vinaigrette.

MEXICAN STUFFED TOMATOES

(serves 2)

4 large tomatoes

¼ green pepper

40 g (2 oz) cooked sweetcorn

40 g (2 oz) medium cheese

lamb's lettuce

1. Wash the tomatoes, cut off the tops and scoop out. Set aside the flesh for a soup.
2. Wash the green pepper, remove the seeds and chop finely.
3. Add the sweetcorn.
4. Cut the cheese into cubes and add to the vegetable mixture. Blend well and fill the tomatoes with the mixture.
5. Arrange the tomatoes on a bed of lettuce.

RAW VEGETABLES WITH DIPS

(serves 2)

1 cucumber
10 radishes
10 mushrooms
3 carrots
cherry tomatoes
dips: yoghurt dressing, aïoli,
   cocktail sauce, Istanbul garlic
   sauce (for recipes see *Dressings
   and Sauces*)

1. Peel the cucumber and cut into strips of approximately 8 cm (3 inches) length.
2. Wash the radishes, cutting off any green parts, leaving 3 cm (1 inch) to make them easy to hold.
3. Rub the mushrooms clean, blanch or steam and let them cool.
4. Peel the carrots and cut into strips of approximately 8 cm (3 inches).
5. Wash the tomatoes, pat dry and put a cocktail stick in each one.
6. Arrange the vegetables on one large dish. Serve with a few dips.

FENNEL SALAD

(serves 2)

2 fennel roots
½ red lettuce
125 ml (¼ pint; ½ cup) olive oil
60 ml (⅛ pint; ¼ cup) wine vinegar
fennel green
basil
oregano
paprika
green stuffed olives

1. Wash the fennel roots. Remove any green parts and save for garnishing. Roughly shred or finely cut the roots.
2. Wash the lettuce, cut into strips and add to the fennel.
3. To make the dressing blend the oil and the vinegar and season with basil, oregano and paprika.
4. Garnish with the green parts from the fennel and green stuffed olives.

SPICY TOMATO SALAD

(serves 2)

4 tomatoes
2 garlic cloves
1 onion
6 black olives
1 tbsp olive oil
fresh basil
dried oregano
salt
pepper

1. Wash the tomatoes, slice and arrange on a large dish.
2. Peel the garlic, slice and divide among the tomatoes.
3. Peel the onion, cut into rings and add to the salad.
4. Garnish with black olives.
5. Pour the olive oil on to the salad and sprinkle with some finely chopped fresh basil and dried oregano. Season with salt and pepper, if necessary.

SOUR STUFFED TOMATOES

(serves 2)

4 tomatoes
4 tbsp pickled vegetables
1 pickled gherkin
1 pickled onion
lettuce

1. Wash the tomatoes, cut off the tops, scoop out the flesh (keep this to make soup) and drain upside down.
2. Mix the pickled vegetables with the pickled gherkin (cut finely) and pickled onions.
3. Fill the tomatoes with this mixture and arrange them on a plate with the lettuce.

GREEN POTATO SALAD

(serves 4)

1 kg (2 lb 4 oz) new potatoes
1 shallot
1 bundle dill
1 bundle parsley
5 sage leaves
1 lemon balm sprig
2 tbsp mayonnaise (see p. 214 for recipe)
1 tbsp sour cream

1. Scrub the potatoes, boil in their skins until cooked. Peel and slice.
2. Peel the shallot and chop.
3. Wash the dill, parsley, sage and lemon balm, pat dry and chop finely or cut.
4. Blend the mayonnaise with the sour cream and mix with the fresh herbs. Blend this sauce with the potato slices.

RAW VEGETABLE SALAD

(serves 1)

¼ Chinese cabbage
¼ cucumber
¼ red pepper
1 tomato
2 tbsp cooked sweetcorn
2 tbsp yoghurt dressing or vinaigrette (see pp. 214–15 for recipes)

1. Wash the Chinese cabbage leaves, pat dry, cut into strips.
2. Peel and slice the cucumber.
3. Cut the red pepper into strips.
4. Cut the tomato into pieces.
5. Mix the cucumber, red pepper and tomato together with the sweetcorn.
6. Add the yoghurt dressing or vinaigrette.

RADISH SALAD

(serves 4)

1 bundle radishes
½ cucumber
6 lettuce leaves
3 tbsp horseradish, creamed

1. Remove the stalks from the radishes, wash and slice.
2. Wash the cucumber and slice.
3. Wash the lettuce, pat dry, cut finely and add to the radishes and cucumber.
4. Add the creamed horseradish and blend well.
5. Serve with a green salad or with bread.

FRUIT PREPARATIONS

TROPICAL MANGO COCKTAIL

(serves 4)

1 ripe mango
6 lychees
1 ripe banana
3 passion fruit
125 ml (¼ pint; ½ cup) of
   double cream

1. Peel the mango, remove the stone and cut into pieces.
2. Peel the lychees, remove the stones and add to the mango pieces.
3. Peel the banana, slice thinly, sprinkle with lemon juice to prevent discoloration and add to the rest.
4. Cut the passion fruit in half. Use a teaspoon to scoop out the flesh and blend with the fruit salad.
5. Beat the cream and serve with the mango cocktail.

STUFFED PINEAPPLE

(serves 2)

1 fresh pineapple
2 ripe pears
2 oranges
1 kiwi fruit
125 ml (¼ pint; ½ cup)
   double cream

1. Cut the pineapple in half (set aside 1 half). Remove the hard core and scoop out using a grapefruit knife. Cut the flesh into bite-sized pieces, peel and put in a bowl.
2. Peel the pears, remove the cores, cut into pieces and add to the pineapple pieces.
3. Peel the oranges until the flesh becomes visible and use a sharp knife to separate the segments.
4. Mix the fruit pieces and fill the hollow part of the pineapple.
5. Serve with cream.
6. Peel the kiwi fruit, slice thinly and garnish the pineapple with it.
7. Beat the cream and serve with the pineapple.

WINTER PINEAPPLE

(serves 2)

1 pineapple
2 apples
2 mandarin oranges
100 g (4 oz; ½ cup) hazelnuts

1. Cut the pineapple in half lengthwise (set aside 1 half). Remove the hard core, scoop out, cut the flesh into pieces, peel and put in a bowl.
2. Peel the apples, remove the cores, cut into pieces and mix with the pineapple pieces.
3. Peel the oranges, separate the segments and put into a bowl. Roughly chop.
4. Mix the fruit salad well and fill the pineapple half with it. Sprinkle with chopped hazelnuts and serve.

CINNAMON APPLES

(serves 2)

4 apples
½ lemon
1 apple
2 tbsp hazelnuts, ground
½ tsp cinnamon

1. Wash the 4 apples, dry and remove the cores using an apple corer, creating a hollow. Steam them.
2. Squeeze the lemon and rub the juice into the apple hollows to prevent discoloration.
3. Roughly shred the single apple, sprinkle with a few drops of lemon juice and blend with the hazelnuts and cinnamon.
4. Fill the apple hollows with the apple and cinnamon mixture and serve.

STUFFED PEAR ON A BED OF STRAWBERRIES

(serves 2)

2 large, ripe pears
lemon juice
10 strawberries
4 passion fruit

1. Peel the pears and cut in half. Remove the cores and sprinkle the pears with lemon juice to prevent discoloration.
2. Wash the strawberries (if unavailable use 2 kiwi fruit), remove the stalks and slice thinly. Arrange the slices overlapping on 4 plates.
3. Cut the passion fruit in half, scoop out the flesh and fill the pear halves with it. Arrange the pears on a bed of strawberries and serve.

CITRUS SALAD

(serves 2)

2 oranges
1 pink grapefruit
2 mandarin oranges
1 bunch black grapes
2 tbsp almond flakes

1. Peel the oranges, separate into segments as described under 'Stuffed pineapple' on p. 158 and put the segments in a bowl.
2. Peel the grapefruit and separate into segments. Put the segments into the same bowl as the oranges. Peel the mandarin oranges and separate into segments. Add to the bowl.
3. Wash the grapes, remove them from their stems, cut in half and remove the seeds (also remove the skin if necessary). Mix the fruit well, divide the salad between 2 bowls and sprinkle with the almond flakes.

FRUIT SALAD

(serves 4)

1 pear
1 orange
1 bunch grapes
½ pineapple
2 tbsp raisins soaked in 2 tbsp
  water
whipped cream

1. Peel the pear, remove the core and cut the flesh into pieces.
2. Thickly peel the orange and separate into segments (as described under 'Stuffed pineapple' on p. 158).
3. Wash the grapes, remove them from their stems, cut in half and remove the seeds.
4. Peel the pineapple, remove the hard core and cut into pieces.
5. Add the soaked raisins and their liquid.
6. Mix all the ingredients and serve with whipped cream.

HONEYDEW MELON COCKTAIL

(serves 2)

1 honeydew melon
1 apple
1 tbsp lemon juice
1 banana
1 mandarin orange
2 tbsp cashew nuts, chopped

1. Cut the melon in half, remove the seeds, creating a hollow.
2. Peel the apple, remove the core, cut in to pieces and sprinkle with lemon juice to prevent discoloration.
3. Also add the banana, cut into slices.
4. Peel the mandarin orange, separate into segments and add to the fruit salad.
5. Mix well and fill the hollow of the melon with the cocktail. Garnish with cashew nuts.

REFRESHING SOUR SUMMER SALAD

(serves 4)

2 peaches
2 plums
4 apricots
2 nectarines
sour cream

1. Wash the peaches, cut in half, remove the stones and cut into pieces.
2. Repeat with plums, apricots and nectarines.
3. Mix the fruit well and serve with sour cream.

LAYERS OF FRUIT SALAD

(serves 4)

1 pomegranate
2 oranges
1 avocado
lemon juice
½ pineapple
2 kiwi fruit
200 g (7 oz) strawberries
1 mango
125 ml (¼ pint; ½ cup) orange juice, freshly squeezed
lemon balm

1. Use a tall glass container or a square vase. Cut the pomegranate in half and remove the seeds.
2. Peel the oranges and separate into segments.
3. Peel the avocado, slice and sprinkle with lemon juice to avoid discoloration.
4. Peel the pineapple, remove the hard core and cut the flesh into pieces.
5. Peel the kiwi fruit and slice.
6. Wash the strawberries, remove the stalks and slice.
7. Peel the mango, remove the stone and slice.
8. Arrange the fruit in layers, starting with a layer of pomegranate, followed by a layer of orange, avocado, pineapple, kiwi fruit, strawberry and mango.
9. Coat the fruit salad with the orange juice and garnish with lemon balm.

FOREST-FRUIT COCKTAIL

(serves 2)

100 g (4 oz) blueberries
100 g (4 oz) raspberries
100 g (4 oz) blackberries
100 g (4 oz) currants
4 tbsp (150 g) quark

1. Wash the fruit, pat dry.
2. Divide the cocktail among 4 bowls and coat with quark.

SWEET AVOCADO SALAD

(serves 2)

1 ripe avocado
1 mango
1 orange
1 kiwi fruit
1 apple
yoghurt dressing (see p. 215 for recipe)

1. Peel the avocado, remove the stone and cut into pieces.
2. Repeat with the mango.
3. Peel the orange and separate into segments as described under 'Stuffed pineapple' on p. 158.
4. Peel the kiwi fruit and slice.
5. Peel the apple, remove the core and cut into pieces.
6. Mix the fruit well and serve with a yoghurt dressing.

STUFFED APRICOTS

(serves 2)

8 fresh apricots
2 dried, soaked apricots
150 g (5 oz) sour cream
8 mint leaves

1. Wash the fresh apricots, cut in half and remove the stones.
2. Drain and chop finely the 2 dried, soaked apricots.
3. Blend the sour cream with the dried apricot pieces.
4. Fill 4 of the apricot halves with the sour cream and use the other 4 halves as a lid.
5. Garnish with mint leaves.

FRIED BANANA WITH GINGER

(serves 4)

4 bananas
2 tbsp safflower oil
1 tsp ginger
20 g (1 oz) strawberries
1 kiwi fruit

1. Peel the bananas.
2. Heat the oil in a pan. Fry the bananas and flavour with ginger.
3. Wash the strawberries, remove the stalks and slice.
4. Arrange the strawberry slices on 4 plates and put the fried bananas on top.
5. Garnish with slices of kiwi fruit.

UGLI-GRAPEFRUIT SALAD WITH THYME HONEY

(serves 4)

1 ugli fruit
1 grapefruit
1 orange
1 mandarin orange
5 kumquats
1 tbsp thyme honey
125 ml (¼ pint; ½ cup) orange
  juice, freshly squeezed
2 tbsp lemon juice
1 tsp thyme

1. Peel the ugli fruit, grapefruit, orange and mandarin orange and separate into segments. Cut the segments into pieces and put in a bowl.
2. Wash the kumquats, slice and add to the citrus fruit.
3. Heat the honey, orange and lemon juices and flavour with thyme. Pour the honey sauce over the citrus salad, let it cool, mix and serve.

SHARON FRUIT SALAD

(serves 2)

2 sharon fruit
1 banana
2 kiwi fruit
4 passion fruit
whipped cream

1. Wash the sharon fruit, dry and cut into pieces.
2. Peel the banana, slice and sprinkle with lemon juice to prevent discoloration.
3. Peel and slice the kiwi fruit.
4. Put all the fruit in a bowl and mix.
5. Cut the passion fruit in half and blend the flesh with the salad.
6. Serve with whipped cream.

PINEAPPLE SALAD WITH COCONUT

(serves 4)

½ pineapple
200 g (7 oz) raspberries
100 g (3.5 oz; ½ cup) raisins
  soaked in 2 tbsp water
1 banana
3 tbsp flaked coconut

1. Peel the pineapple, remove the hard core and cut into pieces.
2. Wash the raspberries, remove the stalks and add to the pineapple pieces.
3. Soak the raisins (the night before). Pour the raisins and their liquid over the salad.
4. Peel the banana, slice and combine with the salad.
5. Sprinkle the coconut over the pineapple salad and serve.

SUMMER FRUITS IN FOREST-FRUIT SAUCE

(serves 4)

400 g (14 oz) forest-fruits
  (e.g. blueberries, blackberries,
  raspberries, strawberries)
2 peaches
2 apricots
4 fresh pineapple slices
2 tbsp blueberries
4 mint leaves
whipped cream

1. Wash the forest-fruits, remove the stalks and purée. Strain the fruit purée. Pour on to 4 dessert plates.
2. Wash the peaches, dry, cut into 4 pieces and slice.
3. Wash the apricots, dry and divide into 4.
4. Arrange the peaches, apricots and pineapple on the forest-fruit sauce.
5. Garnish with blueberries, mint and whipped cream.

AVOCADO MOUSSE

(serves 4)

2 ripe avocados
1 grapefruit
3 tbsp whipped cream
lemon balm leaves

1. Cut the avocados in half, remove the stones and scoop out the flesh with a small spoon.
2. Purée the avocado flesh with the juice of half of the grapefruit until smooth and creamy.
3. Blend with the whipped cream and fill the avocado halves with it. Garnish with grapefruit slices from the remaining half and lemon balm leaves.

FIG COCKTAIL

(serves 2)

5 fresh figs
2 peaches
1 banana
lemon juice
125 ml (¼ pint; ½ cup)
  whipped cream
1 tbsp lemon juice
1 tbsp washed grated lemon peel
fresh lemon balm

1. Wash the figs and cut into 4 pieces.
2. Wash the peaches, cut in half, remove the stones and slice.
3. Peel the banana, slice and sprinkle with lemon juice to avoid discoloration. Mix the fruit well.
4. Blend the whipped cream with the lemon juice and peel. Divide the fig cocktail between 2 plates. Put the lemon cream on top.
5. Garnish with lemon balm.

MELON COCKTAIL WITH MINT

(serves 4)

3 tbsp mint leaves, chopped
125 ml (¼ pint; ½ cup) water
1 tbsp honey
1 lemon
1 orange
1 honeydew melon
6 whole mint leaves

1. Put the chopped mint leaves in a small bowl.
2. Blend the water and honey and let this mixture boil gently for 5 minutes. Pour it over the chopped mint leaves, let it cool and then strain.
3. Add the juice of the lemon and orange.
4. Scoop out the melon using a melon scoop.
5. Fill 4 cocktail glasses with the melon and coat with the mint syrup.
6. Garnish with mint leaves.

BANANA–LEMON BALM PURÉE WITH STRAWBERRIES

(serves 4)

2 bananas
½ lemon
8 lemon balm leaves
125 g (5 oz) strawberries
whipped cream

1. Peel the bananas and purée. Add the juice of half a lemon.
2. Wash the lemon balm, pat dry, chop half the leaves finely and blend with the banana purée.
3. Wash the strawberries, pat dry, remove the stalks and slice.
4. Arrange the strawberries and the banana purée on 4 dessert plates.
5. Garnish with whipped cream and the rest of the lemon balm leaves.

APPLE SAUCE WITH SPICY RASPBERRY TOPPING

(serves 4)

6 apples
½ lemon
100 g (4 oz) raspberries
¼ tsp ginger
¼ tsp vanilla powder
¼ tsp nutmeg
4 mint leaves

1. Peel the apples, remove the cores and shred finely. Add the juice of half a lemon to prevent discoloration.
2. Wash the raspberries, remove the stalks (except for the stalks of the 4 raspberries that will serve as decoration) and purée.
3. Flavour the topping with ginger, vanilla and nutmeg.
4. Divide the apple among 4 small bowls and pour some topping on it.
5. Garnish with the 4 raspberries and mint leaves.

BLANCHED PEARS WITH MARJORAM

(serves 4)

4 pears
125 ml (¼ pint; ½ cup) grape or apple juice
2 tbsp lemon juice
2 marjoram sprigs

1. Peel the pears, cut in half, remove the cores.
2. Heat the grape or apple juice, lemon juice and marjoram and blanch the pears in it.
3. Serve hot or cold.

APPLE COCKTAIL

(serves 4)

2 apples
125 ml (¼ pint; ½ cup) fresh
  orange juice
6 apricots
½ tsp ginger
whipped cream
½ tsp cinnamon

1. Peel the apples, remove the cores and cut into strips.
2. Coat the apples with orange juice.
3. Wash the apricots, cut into 4 pieces, remove the stones and add to the apple pieces.
4. Flavour this cocktail with ginger.
5. Serve the salad in 4 cocktail glasses and garnish with whipped cream and cinnamon.

STONE FRUIT SALAD WITH CINNAMON

(serves 4)

2 peaches
6 apricots
4 plums
2 nectarines
1 orange
½ tsp cinnamon

1. Wash the fruit.
2. Cut all the fruit into 4 pieces, remove the stones and put in a bowl.
3. Pour the juice of the orange on to the fruit, add the cinnamon and mix the salad well.

WARM DISHES

STEAMED VEGETABLES

(serves 4)

1 broccoli
½ small cauliflower
4 carrots
1 tbsp butter
1 tbsp flour
180 ml (⅓ pint; ¾ cup) vegetable stock (see p. 126 for recipe)
60 ml (⅛ pint; ¼ cup) cream
nutmeg
pepper
paprika

1. Wash the broccoli, peel the stems and cut into pieces. Separate the rest into florets.
2. Separate the cauliflower into florets and wash thoroughly.
3. Peel and slice the carrots or cut into strips.
4. Steam the vegetables.
5. To prepare the sauce, heat the butter until melted, add the flour, stirring constantly. When the flour has been absorbed by the butter, add the stock while stirring and simmer until the sauce has thickened. Then add the cream.
6. Season the sauce with nutmeg, pepper and paprika.
7. Serve the warm vegetables with the sauce and boiled potatoes.

CHINESE CABBAGE AU GRATIN

(serves 4)

1 Chinese cabbage
½ tsp stock granules or bouillon powder
200 g (7 oz) mushrooms
1 tbsp butter
grated gruyère or emmental cheese

1. Cut the Chinese cabbage into 4 pieces, wash thoroughly, boil in ample water with stock granules for about 8 minutes and drain. Put the Chinese cabbage pieces in a greased oven dish.
2. Rub the mushrooms clean, slice and stew in butter.
3. Spread the mushrooms over the Chinese cabbage and sprinkle liberally with the cheese.
4. Grill the cabbage dish and serve with a salad.

STUFFED PEPPER

(serves 4)

6 large red or yellow peppers
300 g (11 oz) rice
1 onion
1 small green pepper
150 g (5.3 oz) mushrooms
1 tbsp oil
paprika
curry powder
pepper
lettuce

1. Wash the red or yellow peppers, cut the top part off, briefly blanch or steam and drain.
2. Boil the rice.
3. Meanwhile, peel and finely chop the onion.
4. Wash the green pepper, remove the seeds and cut finely.
5. Rub the mushrooms clean and slice.
6. Heat the oil and sauté the onion, add the green pepper, the mushrooms and the boiled rice and season with paprika, curry powder and pepper.
7. Fill the red or yellow peppers with the rice mixture and put on a heat-resistant oven dish with a lid. Let the peppers heat up in a hot oven for 15 minutes.
8. Serve with the fresh lettuce.

RATATOUILLE

(serves 4)

1 courgette (zuccini)
250 g (9 oz) mushrooms
1 red pepper
1 large onion
2 garlic cloves
5 or 6 beefsteak tomatoes
1 tbsp olive oil
2 bay leaves
½ tbsp stock granules or
   bouillon powder

1. Wash the courgette and slice or cut into pieces.
2. Rub the mushrooms clean, remove the lower part of the stalks and cut in half.
3. Wash the red pepper, remove the seeds and cut into pieces.
4. Peel the onion and cut into rings.
5. Peel the garlic cloves and cut in half.
6. Peel the tomatoes and cut into pieces.
7. Heat the olive oil and sauté the onion rings, adding the rest of the vegetables and mushrooms.
8. Add bay leaves and stock granules. Simmer the vegetables on a low heat until ready.

STEAMED CAULIFLOWER WITH HERB SAUCE

(serves 4)

1 large cauliflower
1 tbsp butter
1 tbsp flour
250 ml (½ pint; 1 cup) vegetable stock (see p. 126 for recipe)
4 tbsp (unsweetened) whipped cream
nutmeg
pepper
1 tbsp fresh parsley, chopped
2 basil leaves, finely shredded

1. Thoroughly wash the cauliflower and steam (separate into florets if preferred).
2. Melt the butter and blend with the flour. When the butter has absorbed the flour completely, add the stock, stirring constantly. Remove the sauce from the heat and blend with the cream. Season with nutmeg, pepper, parsley and basil.
3. Serve with boiled or steamed potatoes.

MIXED VEGETABLES FROM THE WOK

(serves 4)

1 onion
1 garlic clove
1 red pepper
½ Chinese cabbage
200 g (7 oz) mushrooms
200 g (7 oz) broccoli
2 tbsp oil
2 tbsp soy sauce
1 tsp ginger
½ tsp paprika
pepper

1. Peel the onion, cut in half and slice.
2. Peel the garlic and cut into 4 pieces.
3. Wash the pepper, remove the seeds and cut into strips. Wash the Chinese cabbage, pat dry and cut into strips.
4. Rub the mushrooms clean and cut in half.
5. Wash the broccoli, separate into florets and cut the stem into pieces.
6. Heat the oil in a wok and fry the onion for 1 minute while stirring. Add the clove of garlic and the pepper strips and fry for 2 minutes while stirring. Add the broccoli and fry for 1 minute while stirring. Fry the Chinese cabbage and the mushrooms for 1 minute. Season the vegetables with soy sauce, ginger, paprika and pepper.
7. Serve with rice.

VEGETABLE STRIPS WITH CORIANDER SAUCE

(serves 4)

100 g (4 oz) carrots
100 g (4 oz) kohlrabi
100 g (4 oz) courgettes (zuccini)
1 spring onion
1 tbsp butter
2 tsp ground coriander
250 ml (½ pint; 1 cup) cream

1. Wash the carrots, kohlrabi and courgettes and use a peeler to cut them into thin strips like tagliatelle. Only use the outermost part of the courgettes, not the seeds.
2. Blanch or steam the vegetable strips for 2 or 3 minutes.
3. Shred the spring onion and fry in the butter.
4. Add the coriander (or another herb) and cream and pour the sauce over the vegetable strips.

CREAMY BRUSSELS SPROUTS WITH CARROT

(serves 4)

800 g (1 lb 14 oz) Brussels sprouts
6 new carrots
125 ml (¼ pint; ½ cup) cream
4 fresh basil leaves, chopped
pepper
paprika

1. Clean the sprouts.
2. Wash or peel the carrots and cut into equal-sized pieces. Steam the carrots and sprouts until ready.
3. Heat the cream and add the chopped basil leaves.
4. Flavour with pepper and paprika and serve with pasta or potatoes.

STEAMED CARROTS WITH COURGETTE AND SAGE

(serves 4)

1 bundle of new carrots
1 courgette (zuccini)
a few sage leaves
1 small onion
1 tbsp butter
125 ml (¼ pint; ½ cup) cream

1. Remove the green parts from the carrots and discard. Wash the carrots.
2. Wash the courgette and cut into slices or cubes. Steam the carrots and courgette.
3. Wash the sage, pat dry and chop finely.
4. Peel the onion and cut finely. Heat the butter and sauté the onion. Add the sage and cream. Pour the dressing on to the steamed hot vegetables and serve with potatoes.

STUFFED CABBAGE ROLLS WITH SPICY RICE

(serves 4)

100 g (4 oz) rice
1 small onion
½ red pepper
1 tbsp butter
1 tsp curry powder
1 savoy cabbage

1. Boil the rice and let it cool.
2. Peel and shred the onion.
3. Wash the pepper and cut finely.
4. Heat the butter and sauté the onion and the pepper. Add the rice and curry powder. Fry the rice for a while and remove from the heat.
5. Remove the outermost leaves from the cabbage, wash them and boil in water for 6 minutes. Drain them.
6. Put a spoonful of rice in the middle of each leaf and roll the leaves.
7. Serve the rolls with the rest of the rice and curry mixture.

BROCCOLI WITH LEEK CREAM SAUCE

(serves 4)

500 g (18 oz) broccoli
1 leek
1 tbsp butter
125 ml (¼ pint; ½ cup) cream
  sauce (see p. 220 for recipe)
curry powder
pepper

1. Wash the broccoli and steam until ready.
2. Remove any green parts from the leek, discard and cut the rest into rings.
3. Heat the butter and stew the leek.
4. Prepare the cream sauce and add the leek to it. Season with curry powder and pepper.
5. Serve the broccoli with the leek cream sauce and potatoes or pasta.

BRUSSELS SPROUTS AND CHERRY TOMATOES IN HERB BUTTER

(serves 2)

300 g (11 oz) Brussels sprouts
200 g (7 oz) cherry tomatoes
1 or 2 tbsp butter with freshly
  chopped herbs

1. Clean the sprouts, wash and cook.
2. Wash and dry the tomatoes.
3. Heat the herb butter and sauté the sprouts and the tomatoes.
4. Serve with a green salad.

STUFFED MUSHROOMS WITH LEEK

(serves 2)

12 large wild mushrooms
1 leek
3 chives
1 tbsp butter
60 ml (⅛ pint; ¼ cup)
 (unsweetened) whipped cream
cayenne pepper
paprika

1. Rub the mushrooms clean and finely chop the stalks. (Reserve the mushroom caps for later in the recipe.)
2. Clean and wash the leek, discarding any green parts.
3. Wash the chives, pat dry and shred.
4. Heat the butter and stew the leek and the mushroom stalks. Add the chives and cream.
5. Mix together with cayenne pepper and paprika.
6. Fill the mushrooms with the leek mixture and grill until brown.
7. Serve with pasta.

AUBERGINE WITH TOMATOES FROM THE OVEN

(serves 4)

3 aubergines (egg plants)
8 beefsteak tomatoes
1 or 2 tbsp olive oil
oregano
basil
Southern salad (see p. 148
 for recipe)

1. Wash the aubergines, slice, sprinkle with salt and strain for 1 hour.
2. Wash the tomatoes and cut into rings.
3. Sauté the aubergines in the olive oil.
4. Arrange the aubergine slices and the tomatoes alternately in an oven dish.
5. Sprinkle with some oregano and basil and heat the dish in a 200° C (400° F, Gas Mark 6) oven for 40 minutes.
6. Serve with a Southern salad.

Aubergine with Tomatoes from the Oven, *see* page 178
Mixed Vegetables from the Wok, *see* page 174

Vegetarian Lasagna, *see* page 194
Pasta with Steamed Vegetables, *see* page 192
Nasi Goreng, *see* page 195

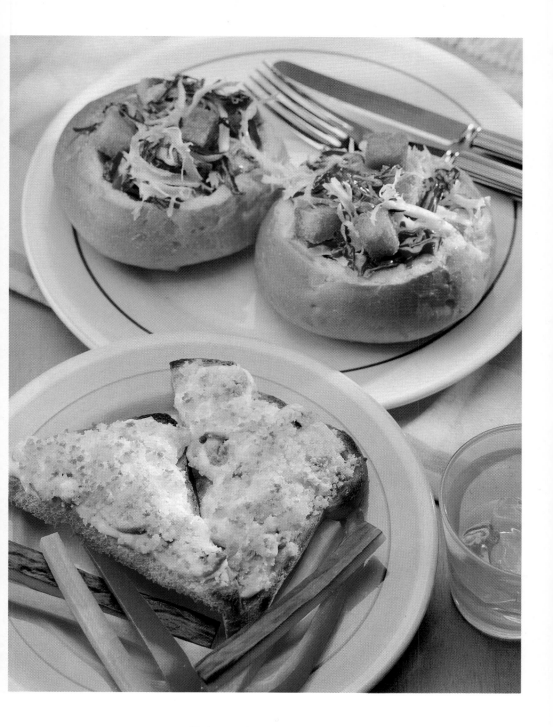

Stuffed Bread Rolls, *see* page 201
Mushroom Toast, *see* page 201

Refreshing Summer Punch, *see* page 226
Rose Hip-Orange Tea, *see* page 226
Apricot Milk, *see* page 225

THREE VEGETABLES IN CHEESE SAUCE

(serves 4)

1 small cauliflower
300 g (11 oz) broccoli
4 carrots
cheese sauce (see p. 220 for recipe)
parsley, chopped

1. Wash the cauliflower and broccoli and separate into florets.
2. Peel the carrots, cut into equal pieces and steam or boil together with the other vegetables.
3. Prepare the cheese sauce and pour it over the vegetables.
4. Sprinkle some parsley over the vegetables.
5. Serve with a green salad.

CREAMY CUCUMBER

(serves 4)

1 shallot
1 cucumber
1 tbsp butter
2 tsp stock granules or bouillon powder
125 ml (¼ pint; ½ cup) cream
cayenne pepper
2 tbsp fresh dill, chopped

1. Peel the shallot and chop finely.
2. Peel the cucumber and cut into equal cubes.
3. Heat the butter and stew the cucumber cubes and shallot.
4. Add the stock granules, stir in the cream. Remove from heat and season with cayenne pepper and dill.
5. Serve with pasta.

KOHLRABI AU GRATIN

(serves 4)

4 kohlrabi
1 small onion
200 g (7 oz) mushrooms
1 tbsp butter
1 garlic clove, minced
pepper
1 tsp stock granules or bouillon
  powder
100 g (4 oz) low-fat grated
  cheese or quark
125 ml (¼ pint; ½ cup) cream

1. Peel the kohlrabi and cut into cubes.
2. Peel the onion and chop finely.
3. Rub the mushrooms clean and slice thinly.
4. Heat the butter and stew the onion, kohlrabi and mushrooms.
5. Add the garlic and season with pepper and stock granules.
6. Combine the cheese and cream with the vegetables.
7. Serve hot with a mixed salad.

STUFFED AUBERGINE

(serves 4)

4 small aubergines (egg plants)
1 shallot
½ red pepper
2 tomatoes
1 tbsp olive oil
1 garlic clove, minced
2 basil leaves, chopped
3 mozzarella cheeses

1. Wash the aubergines, cut in half and scoop out the flesh. Cut the flesh into pieces.
2. Peel the shallot and chop finely.
3. Wash the pepper, remove the seeds and cut finely.
4. Skin the tomatoes and cut into pieces.
5. Heat the olive oil and stew the shallot, the aubergine flesh, the pepper and the tomato. Add the garlic.
6. Remove from heat and add the basil.
7. Fill the aubergine halves with the vegetable mixture and put in to a greased oven dish. Slice the mozzarella cheese (using an egg slicer) and spread over the aubergines. Put the dish in a 180°C (350° F, Gas Mark 4) oven for 40 minutes until ready.

STEAMED VEGETABLE DISH

(serves 2)

2 fennel roots
½ red pepper
½ yellow pepper
1 onion
3 carrots
1 bay leaf
1 tbsp stock granules or bouillon powder
2 or 3 tbsp butter with freshly chopped herbs

1. Cut the fennel into 4 pieces and wash.
2. Wash the peppers, remove the seeds and cut into large pieces.
3. Peel the onion and carrots and slice or cut into large pieces.
4. Put the vegetables into a steaming basket. Add the bay leaf to the water. Steam the vegetables.
5. Put the vegetables on to a dish and spread with herb butter.
6. Serve with potatoes.

ASPARAGUS

(serves 2 to 3)

2 bundles asparagus (green and/or white)
2 parsley sprigs
2 tbsp butter
125 ml (¼ pint; ½ cup) (unsweetened) whipped cream
cayenne pepper

1. Peel the asparagus and steam.
2. Wash the parsley, pat dry and chop finely.
3. Heat the butter until melted, stir in the cream and season with cayenne pepper.
4. Serve with potato puffs (see recipe on p. 184) or new potatoes.

ENDIVE IN PASTRIES

(serves 4)

1 large head of endive
butter
125 ml (¼ pint; ½ cup) cream
  sauce (for recipe see p. 220)
1 garlic clove, minced
stock granules or bouillon powder
nutmeg
4 puff pastry cases

1. Wash the endive and boil down adding a little butter.
2. Remove from heat and add the cream sauce.
3. Season with garlic, stock granules and nutmeg. Fill puff pastry cases with the endive mixture and heat them up in a hot oven.

FRIED VEGETABLES

(serves 4)

1 shallot
½ red pepper
200 g (7 oz) broccoli
100 g (4 oz) mushrooms
2 tbsp butter
pepper
paprika
curry powder

1. Peel the shallot and cut finely.
2. Wash the pepper, remove the seeds and cut finely.
3. Wash the broccoli, drain and cut into pieces.
4. Rub the mushrooms clean and slice.
5. Heat the butter and sauté the vegetables. Season with pepper, curry powder and paprika.
6. Serve with mashed potato or rice.

POTATO DISHES

MASHED POTATO

(serves 4)

1 kg (2 lb 4 oz) potatoes
⅛ litre (¼ pint; ½ cup) cream
⅛ litre (¼ pint; ½ cup) vegetable
  stock (see p. 126 for recipe)
25 g (1 oz) butter
nutmeg
mace
pepper

1. Peel the potatoes, boil them and then pour off the water.
2. Add the cream, stock and butter and purée using a masher or blender. Season with nutmeg, mace and pepper.

POTATO PUFFS

For potato puffs, make sure the mashed potato is slightly thicker and use a piping bag to squirt the puffs on to a baking tray. Grill until golden brown.

POTATO AU GRATIN

(serves 2)

500 g (18 oz) potatoes
1 garlic clove
125 ml (¼ pint; ½ cup) cream
pepper
100 g (3.5 oz; ½ cup)
  breadcrumbs

1. Peel the potatoes and slice thinly (using a food processor). Steam the potato slices but not for too long or else they will fall apart.
2. Grease a shallow oven dish and rub with garlic. Arrange the potato slices on the dish and coat with cream. Sprinkle with pepper and breadcrumbs.
3. Grill the potatoes until they develop a brown crust.

OVEN CHIPS/FRENCH FRIES

(serves 4)

6 large, firm potatoes
paprika
salt
pepper
4 tbsp oil

1. Peel the potatoes, cut into chips/French fries and spread out on a greased baking tray. Sprinkle with paprika and, if required, salt and pepper.
2. Pour the oil on to the chips/French fries, cover with aluminium foil and bake in a preheated oven at 220° C (425° F, Gas Mark 7) for 30 minutes. Remove the foil and bake the chips/french fries for another 15 minutes or until golden brown. Every now and then, turn them over.

POTATO SKINS WITH SOUR CREAM

(serves 2)

4 large, new potatoes
butter
herbs
sour cream
chives

1. Scrub the potatoes, boil and then pour off the water. Cut the potatoes lengthwise into 4 pieces. Cut out the flesh with a sharp knife, but leave ½ cm of flesh in the skin.
2. Arrange the potato skins on a greased baking tray and coat with the melted butter. Sprinkle with herbs and bake for 15–20 minutes in a 230° C (450° F, Gas Mark 8) oven until crisp.
3. Serve the potato skins lukewarm or warm with sour cream and chives and a salad.

STEWED POTATOES

(serves 4)

1 kg (2 lb 4 oz) potatoes
1 onion
1 tbsp butter
1 bay leaf
pepper
stock granules or bouillon powder

1. Peel the potatoes and cut into cubes.
2. Peel the onion and cut finely.
3. Heat the butter and stew the potatoes and the onions on a low heat. Add the bay leaf and season with pepper and stock granules.

HOTCHPOTCH

(serves 4)

mashed potato (see recipe on p. 184)
selection of vegetables

1. Blend the mashed potato (made from 1 kg of potatoes) with boiled, steamed or raw vegetables (e.g. carrots, cauliflower, spinach).
2. Serve the hotchpotch with a refreshing salad.

POTATO RÖSTI

(serves 4)

4 large potatoes
1 tbsp butter
salt
pepper

1. Peel the potatoes and shred roughly (using a food processor). Squeeze out the shredded potato on to a clean kitchen towel or colander, draining the liquid.
2. Heat the butter in a pan. Put the potatoes in the pan and slightly mash with a fork, creating a cake. Sprinkle with salt and pepper. Fry until the bottom turns golden brown, then turn over and fry the other side until golden brown and serve.

POTATO SALAD

(serves 1)

3 medium-sized potatoes
½ onion or shallot
a few chives
1 parsley sprig
¼ celeriac
2 carrots
lamb's lettuce

1. Boil the potatoes in their skins, let them cool, peel and cut into cubes.
2. Peel the onion or shallot and chop.
3. Wash the chives and parsley, pat dry, chop finely and blend with the potato cubes.
4. Peel and roughly shred the celeriac and carrots.
5. Blend the shredded vegetables with the potato cubes and garnish with a few leaves of lettuce.

(See also recipe on p. 139.)

POTATOES WITH HERB BUTTER

(serves 4)

1 kg (2 lb 4 oz) potatoes
butter with freshly chopped herbs

1. Boil the potatoes with or without their skins.
2. Put some herb butter in between the hot potatoes and let the butter melt.
3. Serve with boiled or steamed vegetables.

POTATO SALAD WITH SOUR CREAM

(serves 4)

500 g (18 oz) potatoes
1 pepper
2 tbsp sour cream
chives

1. Boil the potatoes in their skins, peel and cut into cubes.
2. Wash the pepper, remove the seeds and mix with the potato cubes. Add the sour cream and garnish with fresh chives.
3. Serve with a salad.

187

POTATO–CELERIAC PURÉE

(serves 4)

500 g (18 oz) potatoes
300 g (11 oz) peeled celeriac
butter
60 ml (⅛ pint; ¼ cup) cream
nutmeg
pepper

1. Peel the potatoes and cook with the celeriac.
2. Pour off the water and add the butter and cream.
3. Purée the vegetables and season with nutmeg and pepper.

HERB PURÉE

(serves 4)

mashed potato (see recipe on p. 184)
3 tbsp fresh herbs, chopped (e.g. chives, parsley, chervil)

1. To the mashed potato (made from 1 kg of potatoes) add the herbs and blend.
2. Serve with steamed vegetables.

PASTA AND RICE DISHES

FRESH PASTA

(serves 2)

200 g (7 oz) durum wheat flour
2 eggs
1 tbsp oil

1. Put the flour in a bowl, make a hole in the middle and add the eggs.
2. Add the oil and knead until elastic. Knead the dough into a ball, cover and set aside for 30 minutes.
3. Divide the dough into equal pieces and roll with a rolling pin or use a pasta maker. Cut the dough into strips, slices or other shapes.
4. Cook the pasta until al dente (cooked but not soft).

(The quantities in the following recipes are for dried pasta. If you use fresh pasta for any of the recipes, you will need approximately twice the weight.)

FINE SPAGHETTI WITH MIXED VEGETABLES

(serves 4)

300 g (11 oz) fine spaghetti
400 g (14 oz) sugar peas
12 baby corncobs
300 g (11 oz) mushrooms
3 spring onions
2 tbsp butter
salt
cayenne pepper
creamy red pepper sauce
 (for recipe see p. 219)

1. Wash the sugar peas and remove the fibrous threads. Wash the corncobs.
2. Rub the mushrooms clean.
3. Remove the roots and any withered green parts from the spring onions. Slice them.
4. Heat the butter and gently stew the mushrooms, baby corncobs and peas. Season with salt and cayenne pepper.
5. Meanwhile, cook the spaghetti and drain. Divide the spaghetti among 4 preheated plates, together with a few spoons of mixed vegetables and mushrooms. Serve with the creamy red pepper sauce.

COLD PASTA SALAD

(serves 1)

100 g (4 oz) mixed pasta
1 broccoli head
a few leaves of iceberg lettuce
1 bundle watercress
2 carrots
2 tbsp mayonnaise (see recipe on p. 214)

1. Cook the pasta until al dente (cooked but not soft) and let it cool.
2. Wash the broccoli and separate into florets. Steam and allow to cool.
3. Wash the lettuce, pat dry and cut into strips.
4. Wash the watercress, pat dry and add to the pasta with the lettuce strips and the broccoli florets.
5. Roughly shred the carrots and mix with the pasta.
6. Add the mayonnaise and mix the salad well.

PASTA WITH HERBS

(serves 4)

500 g (18 oz) pasta
4 tbsp olive oil
2 tbsp basil or parsley, chopped

1. Cook the pasta until al dente (cooked but not soft).
2. Heat the oil and pour over the pasta.
3. Sprinkle with basil or parsley.

PASTA WITH STEAMED VEGETABLES

(serves 4)

1 small courgette (zuccini)
3 new carrots
300 g (11 oz) fresh peas
3 spring onions
400 g (14 oz) pasta
½ onion
1 tbsp butter
250 ml (½ pint; 1 cup) cream
saffron threads
salt
pepper
fresh thyme

1. Wash the courgette and carrots and cut into equal pieces.
2. Wash the fresh peas and remove any fibrous threads.
3. Wash and remove the roots from the spring onions, cut the green parts into 2 pieces and the onions into 4 pieces.
4. Put the vegetables in a steamer.
5. Meanwhile, cook the pasta until al dente (cooked but not soft) and drain.
6. Peel the onion and sauté in the butter.
7. Add the cream with the saffron threads. Add salt and pepper if required.
8. Pour the cream sauce over the vegetables and serve the pasta and the vegetables in 2 separate bowls.
9. Garnish with thyme.

THREE-COLOUR PASTA WITH LEEK SAUCE

(serves 4)

3 leeks
200 g (7 oz) mushrooms
500–600 g (18–21 oz) of three-colour pasta
1 tbsp butter
curry powder
pepper
stock granules or bouillon powder
250 ml (½ pint; 1 cup) cream

1. Cut off the roots and any green parts from the leeks (use the green parts for a soup). Cut the leeks in half, wash thoroughly and cut into rings.
2. Rub the mushrooms clean. Remove the lower part of the stalks and slice.
3. Boil the pasta until al dente (cooked but not soft).
4. Meanwhile, heat the butter and stew the leek and the mushrooms. Season with curry powder, pepper and stock granules.
5. Add the cream, stir well and pour over the pasta.
6. Serve with a salad.

REFRESHING PASTA SALAD

(serves 1)

100 g (4 oz) butterfly pasta

1 carrot

1 bundle mustard and cress

2 tbsp beansprouts

herb mayonnaise (see p. 215 for recipe)

1. Boil the pasta until al dente (cooked but not soft) and let it cool.
2. Peel the carrot, shred it and add to the pasta.
3. Wash the mustard and cress and mix with the pasta. Add the beansprouts and mix the salad well.
4. Blend the salad well and coat with the herb mayonnaise.

TAGLIATELLE WITH OYSTER MUSHROOMS

(serves 4)

1 kg (2 lb 4 oz) oyster mushrooms

1 shallot

1 tbsp butter

1 tbsp olive oil

2 garlic cloves, minced

cayenne pepper

400–500 g (14–18 oz) tagliatelle

250 ml (½ pint; 1 cup) (unsweetened) whipped cream

6 fresh basil leaves

1. Rub the mushrooms clean.
2. Peel the shallot and chop finely.
3. Fry the mushrooms and the shallot in butter and olive oil and flavour with garlic and cayenne pepper.
4. Meanwhile, cook the pasta until al dente (cooked but not soft), drain and blend with the mushrooms. Add the cream.
5. Garnish with basil.

VEGETARIAN LASAGNA

(serves 4)

450 g (16 oz) broccoli
stock granules or bouillon powder
salt
pepper
1 endive
2 tbsp butter
200 g (7 oz) mushrooms
250 ml (½ pint; 1 cup) cream
500 g (18 oz) lasagna
3 tbsp breadcrumbs

1. Wash the broccoli, divide into florets, cut the stalks into pieces and cook. Purée the broccoli and season with stock granules, salt and pepper.
2. Wash the endive and cook it in the butter. Season.
3. Rub the mushrooms clean, slice and fry in butter.
4. Stir some of the cream into the broccoli purée and some into the endive mixture.
5. Meanwhile, cook the lasagna.
6. Grease a square oven dish and cover the bottom with some of the lasagna strips. Pour a layer of broccoli sauce on to the lasagna. Then put the next layer of lasagna on top, followed by the fried mushrooms, another layer of lasagna and the endive mixture. Continue doing this until the sauces, lasagna and mushrooms have been used up. Make sure the final layer is endive.
7. Sprinkle with breadcrumbs and grill until heated through.

FRIED RICE

(to use up left-over boiled rice)

boiled rice
1 tbsp oil
garlic
ginger
curry powder

1. Fry the boiled rice briefly in oil and season with garlic, ginger and curry powder.
2. Serve with oriental vegetable dishes.

NASI GORENG

(serves 4)

300 g (11 oz) rice
1 small onion
1 garlic clove
1 large carrot
1 leek
½ red pepper
200 g (7 oz) fresh peas
150 g (5 oz) mushrooms
1 tbsp oil
1 tbsp soy sauce
½ tsp paprika
¼ tsp curry powder
¼ tsp ginger
fresh chives, chopped

1. Cook the rice.
2. Peel and chop the onion finely and mince the garlic.
3. Peel the carrot and cut finely.
4. Wash the leek and red pepper and cut finely.
5. Cook the peas.
6. Rub the mushrooms clean and slice thinly.
7. Heat the oil in a wok and fry everything together, stirring constantly for 5 minutes.
8. Season with soy sauce. Add the rice and mix with the vegetables. Flavour with paprika, curry powder and ginger.
9. Garnish with chives.

SPICY PEPPER RICE

(serves 4)

200 g (7 oz) rice
1 red pepper
1 green pepper
½ onion
½ tbsp oil
1 garlic clove, minced
2 drops tabasco
½ tsp curry powder

1. Cook the rice.
2. Wash the red and green peppers, remove the seeds and cut finely.
3. Peel the onion and chop finely.
4. Heat the oil and fry the onion and the peppers.
5. Add the garlic and rice. Mix the rice and the vegetables well. Add tabasco and curry powder. Serve as a side-dish.

RISOTTO WITH FUNGI

(serves 4)

250 g (9 oz) rice
1 shallot
1 garlic clove
1 kg (2 lb 4 oz) mixed fungi
(e.g. oyster mushrooms,
chanterelles, Parisian
mushrooms, morels, ceps)
2 tbsp butter
pepper
250 ml (½ pint; 1 cup) cream
fresh basil leaves
fresh oregano

1. Cook the rice.
2. Peel the shallot and garlic and chop finely.
3. Rub the fungi clean, slice the large ones and leave the small ones whole.
4. Fry the fungi in butter with the shallot and garlic. Season with pepper.
5. Mix the rice with the mixed fungi and add the cream. Season the risotto with basil and oregano.

MIXED RICE

(serves 4)

150 g (5 oz) rice
50 g (2 oz) wild rice
1 shallot
1 tbsp butter
paprika
pepper
chives, chopped

1. Cook both types of rice separately.
2. Peel the shallot, shred and fry in butter.
3. Add the rice and season with paprika and pepper.
4. Garnish with chives and serve as a side-dish.

COLD RICE SALAD

(serves 4)

150 g (5 oz) rice
½ red pepper
1 spring onion
3 tbsp freshly cooked green peas
3 tbsp cooked sweetcorn
3 tbsp mayonnaise (see p. 214 for recipe)

1. Cook the rice.
2. Wash the pepper, remove the seeds and chop finely.
3. Peel the sping onion, chop finely and blend with the rice and pepper.
4. Mix the peas and sweetcorn with the rice salad. Add the mayonnaise and mix well.
5. Serve with a green salad.

BREAD ROLLS
AND TOASTS

RAW VEGETABLE BREAD ROLLS

(serves 1)

2 bread rolls

2 tbsp mayonnaise (see p. 214 for recipe)

4 lettuce leaves

¼ cucumber

2 tbsp carrots, shredded

1 bundle mustard and cress

6 radishes

chives, chopped

1. Cut the bread rolls in half and spread with the mayonnaise.
2. Wash the lettuce, pat dry and divide between the bread rolls.
3. Peel the cucumber, slice and put on the bread rolls with the carrots and mustard and cress.
4. Wash the radishes, remove any green parts and slice. Use them to garnish the bread rolls and scatter some finely chopped chives on top.

AVOCADO BREAD ROLL

(serves 1)

2 bread rolls

4 lettuce leaves

4 radishes

¼ cucumber

1 bundle mustard and cress

1 avocado

1 tbsp lemon juice

½ tsp curry powder

1. Cut the bread rolls in half.
2. Wash the lettuce, pat dry and cut in strips.
3. Wash the radishes, remove the stalks and slice.
4. Peel the cucumber and slice.
5. Wash the mustard and cress and pat dry.
6. Peel the avocado, cut in half, remove the stone and purée the flesh. Add lemon juice and season with curry powder.
7. Spread the avocado purée on the bread rolls and garnish with the lettuce strips, the radish slices, the cucumber slices and the mustard and cress.

STUFFED BREAD ROLLS

(serves 1)

2 round bread rolls
2 curly endive leaves
1 piece red cabbage
½–1 tbsp herb mayonnaise
(see p. 214 for recipe)
butter

1. Slice the top off each bread roll, scoop out the contents and cut into cubes.
2. Wash the endive, pat dry, cut finely and put into a bowl.
3. Shred the red cabbage and add to the endive. Add the herb mayonnaise and mix well.
4. Fry the bread cubes in a little butter until golden brown and add to the salad.
5. Fill the bread rolls with the salad.

MUSHROOM TOAST

(serves 4)

4 slices bread
200 g (7 oz) mushrooms
1 tbsp butter
125 ml (¼ pint; ½ cup) cream
sauce (for recipe see p. 220)
nutmeg
paprika
stock granules or bouillon powder
pepper
2 tbsp breadcrumbs

1. Toast the bread.
2. Rub the mushrooms clean and slice.
3. Heat the butter and stew the mushrooms.
4. Stir in the mushrooms into the cream sauce and season with nutmeg, paprika, stock granules and pepper. Add some cornflour paste (cornflour mixed with water) to the sauce to thicken if necessary.
5. Spread a thick layer of the mushroom sauce over the toasted bread and sprinkle with the breadcrumbs.
6. Put the toasted bread under the grill until brown. Arrange on plates, decorated with raw vegetables.

TOAST WITH SCRAMBLED EGGS

(serves 4)

4 slices bread
4 egg yolks
4 tbsp water
salt
pepper
1 parsley sprig
4 chive blades
2 basil leaves
4 oregano leaves
1 tbsp butter

1. Toast the bread.
2. Beat the egg yolks and water in a bowl and add salt and pepper.
3. Finely chop the herbs and stir into the beaten eggs.
4. Melt the butter in a pan, add the eggs and let them set while stirring.
5. Put the scrambled eggs on the toasted bread and arrange on 4 plates.

STUFFED BREAD ROLLS WITH LEEK RAGOÛT

(serves 4)

4 round crusty bread rolls
1 leek
150 g (5 oz) mushrooms
6 cooked asparagus spears
2 tbsp butter
125 ml (¼ pint; ½ cup)
  (unsweetened) whipped cream
pepper
stock granules or bouillon powder

1. Slice the top off each bread roll, scoop out the contents and cut into cubes to fry afterwards in some of the butter (croûtons).
2. Grill the bread rolls briefly until crusty.
3. Clean the leek, discarding any roots and green parts and cut into rings.
4. Rub the mushrooms clean and slice.
5. Cut the asparagus into pieces.
6. Heat the rest of the butter and stew the leek rings and the mushroom slices. Add the asparagus pieces.
7. Mix with the cream and season with pepper and stock granules.
8. Fill the toasted rolls with the ragoût, sprinkle them with the croûtons and serve with raw vegetables and any remaining sauce.

SPICY BREAD CROÛTONS

(serves 4)

2 slices bread
1 tbsp butter
1 tbsp olive oil
1 garlic clove, minced
2 tbsp fresh herbs, chopped

1. Remove the crusts from the bread, discard and cut the bread into cubes.
2. Heat the butter and olive oil and fry the bread cubes until crusty.
3. Add the garlic and herbs.
4. Serve these croûtons with a salad or soup.

BREAD ROLLS WITH FRIED PEPPER

(serves 2)

2 bread rolls
1 red pepper
1 tbsp oil
1 garlic clove, minced
2 curly endive leaves

1. Cut the bread rolls in half.
2. Wash the pepper, remove the seeds and cut into strips.
3. Heat the oil and fry the pepper strips with the garlic.
4. Put the endive on the bread rolls, together with the pepper strips.

OYSTER MUSHROOM BUNS

(serves 2)

2 round bread rolls

200 g (7 oz) oyster mushrooms

1 tbsp butter

1 garlic clove, minced

2 lettuce leaves

1 tbsp mayonnaise (see p. 214 for recipe)

1 tbsp (unsweetened) whipped cream

fresh herbs

salt

pepper

1. Cut the bread rolls in half.
2. Rub the mushrooms clean and fry in butter with the garlic.
3. Put the lettuce and mushrooms on the rolls.
4. Mix the mayonnaise with the cream, herbs, salt and pepper.
5. Put a spoonful of this sauce on each bread roll.

CHEESE DISHES

CHEESE SALAD

(serves 1)

100 g (3.5 oz) cheese
  (e.g. vegetarian cheese,
  camembert, gouda, brie)
mixed lettuce
4 lamb's lettuce florets
1 tomato
1 chicory spear
chives
radish
100 g (3.5 oz) fresh low-fat
  soft cheese
fresh herbs, chopped

1. Wash the mixed and lamb's lettuces and pat dry.
2. Wash the tomato and cut into pieces.
3. Cut the chicory in half, remove the bitter core and cut finely.
4. Mix the vegetables together and garnish with chives and the radish.
5. Serve with the cheese, accompanied by a dressing of soft cheese mixed with herbs.

STUFFED MUSHROOMS

(serves 4)

20 medium-sized mushrooms
200 g (7 oz) quark
1 tbsp cheese, grated
1 garlic clove, minced
parsley
chives
2 basil leaves
pepper
paprika

1. Rub the mushrooms clean, remove the stalks and set aside for another dish.
2. Blend the quark with the cheese and garlic. Season this mixture with the finely chopped herbs, pepper and paprika.
3. Fill the mushroom buttons with the quark mixture and place under the grill until brown.

(You could also use small tomatoes instead of the mushrooms. An alternative recipe for Stuffed Mushrooms appears on p. 118.)

FRUITY CHEESE STICKS

(snack or appetizer for 4)

4 pieces cheese of your choice (camembert, gouda, brie, cheddar)

2 kiwi fruit

1 bunch black grapes

2 mandarin oranges

8 skewers

1. Cut the cheese into equal cubes.
2. Peel the kiwi fruit and cut into cubes.
3. Wash the grapes and remove from their stems.
4. Peel the mandarin oranges and separate into segments.
5. Arrange cheese and fruit cubes alternately on the skewers.

MUSHROOMS IN BOURSIN

(serves 4)

500 g (18 oz) mushrooms

1 tbsp butter

1 packet Boursin

1 garlic clove, minced

1. Rub the mushrooms clean and slice thinly.
2. Stew the mushrooms in butter. Add the Boursin (or another herb cream cheese) and garlic. Heat until the cheese has melted.
3. Serve with a salad.

STUFFED CHERRY TOMATOES

(serves 4)

12 or 16 cherry tomatoes
150 g (5 oz) cream cheese
chives
celery salt
mustard and cress
a few lettuce leaves

1. Wash and dry the tomatoes. Cut off the tops and scoop out the flesh using a sharp knife.
2. Mix the cream cheese with the finely chopped chives and celery salt.
3. Fill the tomatoes with this mixture and garnish the plate with mustard and cress and lettuce.

TOMATOES COVERED WITH CHEESE

(serves 4)

5 tomatoes
2 mozzarella cheeses
salt
pepper
5 basil leaves

1. Wash the tomatoes, dry, remove the stalks and slice.
2. Slice the mozzarella cheese (using an egg slicer).
3. Put the cheese and tomato slices alternately into a greased oven dish. Sprinkle with some salt and pepper and grill until the cheese has melted.
4. Wash the basil, pat dry, cut finely and scatter over the hot dish.

STUFFED FENNEL ROOTS

(serves 2 to 3)

4 large fennel roots
½ red pepper
1 shallot
1 tbsp butter
1 garlic clove, minced
gruyère cheese, grated

1. Wash the fennel, remove the brown spots and steam. Use a teaspoon to make a hole in the roots and then cut the scooped out flesh into pieces.
2. Wash the pepper, remove the seeds and cut the flesh into pieces.
3. Peel the shallot and chop finely.
4. Heat the butter and stew the pepper, the onion and the fennel. Season with garlic.
5. Fill the fennel roots with the vegetable mixture and sprinkle some cheese on top. Grill until the cheese has melted.

STUFFED GOAT'S CHEESE

(appetizer for 4)

4 fresh goat's cheeses (75 g, 3 oz each)
150 g (5 oz) cream cheese
1 tbsp fresh basil leaves, chopped
1 parsley sprig, chopped
3 chives
watercress

1. Cut the goat's cheeses in half horizontally.
2. Mix the cream cheese with the basil, parsley and chives.
3. Spread the cream cheese mixture over 4 of the goat's cheese halves. Put the remaining halves on top. Garnish with a bed of watercress.

GOAT'S CHEESE AU GRATIN

(appetizer for 4)

4 goat's cheeses
curly endive
lamb's lettuce
tomato
cucumber

1. Grill the goat's cheeses briefly.
2. Serve them on a bed of endive, lamb's lettuce, tomato and cucumber.

PEAR WITH GOAT'S CHEESE

(appetizer for 4)

2 pears
150 g (5 oz) goat's cheese
100 g (3.5 oz) cream cheese
pepper
4 mint leaves

1. Peel the pears, remove the cores, slice and arrange on 4 plates.
2. Cut off the rind from the goat's cheese, flatten the cheese with a fork, stir in the cream cheese and season with pepper.
3. With cool hands, roll the cheese into a sausage shape, and cut into 12 equal slices.
4. Divide the cheese slices among the 4 plates and garnish with mint.

GORGONZOLA MUSHROOMS

(serves 4)

250 g (9 oz) mushrooms
150 g (5 oz) gorgonzola
fresh chives

1. Rub the mushrooms clean, remove the stalks and set them aside for another dish.
2. Flatten the gorgonzola with a fork and fill the mushroom buttons with it.
3. Put the mushroom buttons on to a greased oven dish, sprinkle with some finely shredded chives and grill until the cheese has melted.

CHEESE DISH

(serves 4)

1 piece brie	1. Arrange the cheeses on a large cheeseboard.
1 piece camembert	2. Garnish with the fruit.
1 piece herb cheese	
1 piece gouda, etc	
3 bunches of grapes	
2 mandarin oranges	
2 kiwi fruit	
3 apricots	

QUARK WITH FOREST-FRUITS

(serves 4)

150 g (5 oz) forest-fruits (raspberries, blackberries, redcurrants ...)
200 g (7 oz) low-fat quark
4 tbsp whipped cream

1. Wash and dry the forest-fruits.
2. Mix the quark with the forest-fruits and decorate with the cream.
3. Garnish with left-over fruits if required.

CHEESE–FRUIT SALAD

(serves 4)

150 g (5 oz) young edam or gouda
1 orange
1 kiwi fruit
1 orange
1 apple

1. Remove the rind from the cheese and cut the cheese into cubes.
2. Peel the orange and separate into segments.
3. Peel the kiwi fruit, cut into pieces and mix with the cheese and orange.
4. Peel the apple, remove the core, cut into pieces and mix with the salad.

DRESSINGS AND SAUCES

MAYONNAISE

1 egg
1 tsp mustard
½ tsp oil (preferably not olive oil)
1 or 2 lemons
salt
pepper

1. In a blender mix together the egg and the mustard.
2. Add the oil little by little. Add the lemon juice and season with salt and pepper.

(If you want to beat the mayonnaise by hand, only use the egg yolk.)

VINAIGRETTE

1 tsp mustard or mustard seed, ground
125 ml (¼ pint; ½ cup) oil
60 ml (⅛ pint; ¼ cup) wine vinegar, cider vinegar or lemon juice
spices
herbs
½ onion

1. Mix the mustard with the oil and vinegar.
2. Season with spices, herbs and finely chopped onion.

TOMATO VINAIGRETTE

1 cup vinaigrette (without onion) (see above for recipe)
2 tbsp tomato ketchup
oregano
paprika

1. Mix the vinaigrette with the tomato ketchup.
2. Season with oregano and paprika.

YOGHURT DRESSING

2 parts mayonnaise (see previous
  page for recipe)
1 part yoghurt or buttermilk
fresh or dried herbs, chopped
onion
garlic

1. Blend the mayonnaise with the yoghurt or
   buttermilk.
2. Season with the herbs, onion and garlic.

HERB MAYONNAISE

2 tbsp mayonnaise (see previous
  page for recipe)
1 tbsp fresh herbs

Blend the mayonnaise with the fresh herbs.

SOUR CREAM

200 g (7 oz) sour cream
fresh garden herbs (e.g. dill,
  chives, parsley, basil,
  peppermint)

Mix the sour cream with the herbs.

SPICY RED SAUCE

125 ml (¼ pint; ½ cup) tomato
  ketchup
1 tbsp horseradish paste
1 tsp French mustard
½ tbsp white wine vinegar
½ tbsp lemon juice
3 drops tabasco
1 spring onion
cayenne pepper
paprika

1. Mix the tomato ketchup, horseradish, mustard, vinegar, lemon juice and tabasco together.
2. Finely cut the spring onion and add to the rest. Blend the sauce well and season with cayenne pepper and paprika.
3. Serve with iceberg lettuce and grilled vegetables.

MUSTARD SAUCE

3 tbsp mustard (with seeds)
2 tbsp mayonnaise (see p. 214
  for recipe)
1 tbsp lemon juice
2 tbsp sour cream
2 lemon balm leaves

1. Mix the mustard, mayonnaise, lemon juice and sour cream together.
2. Finely cut the lemon balm and add to the sauce.
3. Serve with boiled or steamed asparagus.

LOUISIANA SALAD DRESSING

3 tbsp home-made aïoli (see below for recipe)

2 tbsp sour cream

2 tbsp tomato ketchup

1 tsp lemon juice

1 tsp spicy mustard

2 spring onions

cayenne pepper

2 drops tabasco

horseradish

salt

1. Mix the aïoli (garlic mayonnaise) with the sour cream, tomato ketchup, lemon juice and mustard.
2. Clean the onions, chop finely and mix with the dressing.
3. Season with cayenne pepper, tabasco, horseradish and salt.
4. Refrigerate for a few hours, before serving with a mixed salad.

AÏOLI (GARLIC MAYONNAISE)

1 tsp mustard

1 egg yolk

250 ml (½ pint; 1 cup) olive oil

½ lemon

2 garlic cloves

1. Prepare a mayonnaise consisting of mustard, egg yolk and olive oil.
2. Add the juice of half a lemon.
3. Squeeze the juice from the garlic over the mayonnaise.
4. Serve with cold potatoes or as a dip.

COCKTAIL SAUCE

4 tbsp mayonnaise (see p. 214 for recipe)
2 tbsp tomato ketchup
1 tsp paprika
pepper

1. Mix the mayonnaise with the tomato ketchup and paprika. Season with pepper.
2. Serve with salads, as a dip, or with cold stuffed tomatoes.

DIET DRESSING

4 beefsteak tomatoes
½ tbsp lemon juice
pepper
fresh basil
oregano

1. Skin the tomatoes, cut into pieces, purée and drain.
2. Mix the tomato purée with lemon juice.
3. Season with pepper, basil and oregano.

ISTANBUL GARLIC SAUCE

4 tbsp mayonnaise (see p. 214 for recipe)
2 tbsp Greek yoghurt
¼ cucumber
2 garlic cloves
salt
pepper
1 tbsp chives, chopped

1. Mix the mayonnaise with the yoghurt.
2. Peel the cucumber, shred and add to the sauce.
3. Peel the garlic and squeeze the juice on to the cucumber.
4. Season with salt and pepper and garnish with chives.

CREAMY RED PEPPER SAUCE

1 tbsp butter or margarine
2 red peppers
125 ml (¼ pint; ½ cup) cream
1 shallot
pepper
salt

1. Chop the peppers and the shallot finely.
2. Fry the peppers and shallot in the butter or margarine until soft.
3. Put the vegetables into a blender together with the cream and season with salt and pepper.
4. Blend until smooth and serve hot.

MEXICAN AVOCADO DIP

2 ripe avocados
3 tbsp lime juice
1 tomato, skinned and deseeded
1 shallot, finely chopped
pepper
tabasco

1. Peel the avocados, remove the stones and cut into pieces.
2. Add the lime juice, tomato and shallot.
3. Purée the ingredients until the sauce becomes smooth. Season with pepper and tabasco and serve as a dip with vegetables and tortillas.

CURRY SAUCE

½ onion
butter
1 tsp curry powder
250 ml (½ pint; 1 cup) vegetable stock (see p. 126 for recipe)
cornflour
water
pepper
paprika
saffron

1. Peel the onion, cut finely and sauté in the butter.
2. Add the curry powder, stirring constantly to prevent burning and then add the stock.
3. Let the sauce heat through and thicken with the cornflour mixed with a little water.
4. Season with pepper, paprika and saffron.

SAUCE PROVENÇAL

½ onion
½ pepper
1 tbsp olive oil
3 beefsteak tomatoes
2 bay leaves
1 pinch oregano
1 pinch basil
1 pinch mixed herbs
1 tsp stock granules or bouillon powder
paprika
pepper

1. Peel the onion and cut finely.
2. Wash the pepper, remove the seeds and cut finely.
3. Heat the olive oil and stew the onion and the pepper.
4. Remove the seeds from the tomatoes, skin them and add to the pepper.
5. Add the herbs and stock granules.
6. Simmer on a low heat and season with paprika and pepper.

CREAM SAUCE

1 oz (25 g) butter or margarine
1 tbsp of flour
125 ml (¼ pint; ½ cup) vegetable stock
125 ml (¼ pint; ½ cup) cream
nutmeg
salt
pepper
paprika

1. Heat the butter or margarine until it has melted.
2. Add the flour while stirring constantly.
3. Add the vegetable stock while stirring until the sauce has thickened.
4. Add the cream and season with nutmeg, salt, pepper and paprika.

CHEESE SAUCE

As recipe for Cream Sauce, but instead of cream use 100 g (3.5 oz) of grated cheese such as cheddar, emmental or gruyère.

TOMATO SAUCE

½ onion
4 beefsteak tomatoes
1 tbsp oil
pepper
stock granules or bouillon powder
fresh basil

1. Peel the onion and cut finely.
2. Cut the tomatoes into pieces.
3. Heat the oil and stew the onion and the tomato. Purée the sauce and strain.
4. Season with pepper, stock granules and basil.

BROCCOLI SAUCE

200 g (7 oz) broccoli
125 ml (¼ pint; ½ cup) cream
pepper
stock granules or bouillon powder

1. Wash the broccoli, cut into pieces and steam.
2. Purée the broccoli.
3. Add the cream and season with pepper and stock granules.

NON-ALCOHOLIC
BEVERAGES

ORANGE–GINGER DRINK

10 oranges
1 grapefruit
½ tsp ginger or fresh ginger, shredded

1. Squeeze the oranges and grapefruit.
2. Add the ginger.
3. Pour the juice into tall glasses and serve.

MELON BOWL

1 medium-sized honeydew melon
¾ litre (1½ pints; 3 cups) water
1 lemon
1 whole cinnamon stick
4 mint leaves
1 tbsp honey

1. Peel the melon, remove the seeds, cut into cubes and put in a large bowl.
2. Boil the water, adding the juice of the lemon, the cinnamon and the mint. Also add honey if required.
3. Pour the warm mixture over the melon and let it cool.

MOROCCAN PEPPERMINT TEA

½ litre (1 pint; 2 cups) boiling water
1 handful fresh peppermint leaves
1 tea bag mint tea
2 tbsp honey

1. Pour the boiling water over the peppermint leaves and tea bag.
2. Leave the tea for a while and then add the honey.

(A refreshing tea for a hot summer day.)

YOGHURT DRINK

150 g (5 oz) raspberries
½ litre (1 pint; 2 cups) yoghurt
whipped cream

1. Purée the raspberries.
2. Drain and mix with the yoghurt.
3. Divide among 4 glasses and use a piping bag to decorate with cream.

BANANA DRINK

2 bananas
250 ml (½ pint; 1 cup) yoghurt
125 ml (¼ pint; ½ cup) cream

1. Peel and purée the bananas.
2. Add the yoghurt and cream.
3. Put in a blender until creamy.

APRICOT MILK

6 apricots, dried
½ litre (1 pint; 2 cups) buttermilk

1. Soak the apricots in water, cut into pieces and add the buttermilk and a tablespoon of the liquid from the apricots.
2. Blend the mixture until creamy.

HIBISCUS PUNCH

½ litre (1 pint; 2 cups)
  boiling water
2 tea bags or hibiscus tea
½ litre (1 pint; 2 cups) apple juice
whipped cream
cinnamon

1. Pour the boiling water over the tea bags. Leave the tea for 5 minutes.
2. Remove the tea bags from the water and add the apple juice.
3. Heat the liquid again and pour into cups.
4. Add some cream to each cup and sprinkle with cinnamon.

ROSE HIP–ORANGE TEA

2 tea bags rose hip tea
1 tea bag orange blossom tea
½ litre (1 pint; 2 cups)
  boiling water
½ orange
honey

1. Leave the tea in the boiling water for a while.
2. Wash the orange and slice. Divide the slices among 4 cups and pour the tea over.
3. Sweeten with honey if necessary.

REFRESHING SUMMER PUNCH

100 g (3.5 oz) forest-fruits
  (raspberries, blackberries,
  redcurrants ...)
4 tbsp crushed ice
freshly squeezed orange juice

1. Wash, purée and sieve the forest-fruits.
2. Divide between 4 glasses.
3. Sprinkle the crushed ice on top.
4. Top up with the fresh orange juice.

EXAMPLES OF MENUS

... FOR ELABORATE DINING

Stuffed mushrooms
Raw vegetable soup
Steamed vegetables

Southern tomatoes
Gazpacho
Gardener's salad

Avocado stuffed with raw vegetables
Creamy cucumber soup
Steamed vegetables

Garlic tomatoes
Corn–cheese salad
Ratatouille

Oyster mushrooms coated with
  breadcrumbs
Leek soup
Refreshing pasta salad

Fennel au gratin
Raw tomato soup
Aubergine with tomatoes from the
  oven

Avocado dip
Mushroom soup
Fine spaghetti with mixed
  vegetables

Cauliflower soup
Potato salad
Green salad

Creamy asparagus soup
Creamy Brussels sprouts with
  carrot
Potatoes

Raw vegetables with dips
Festive cream soup
Potato puffs with steamed
  vegetables

Celeriac soup
Steamed cauliflower with herb
  dressing
Potatoes

Avocado soup
Fried vegetables
Rice

Pumpkin soup
Stuffed cabbage rolls with spicy rice

Chinese vegetable soup
Mixed vegetables from the wok
Nasi Goreng

Fine herb cream soup
Fine asparagus salad
Vegetable tagliatelle with coriander
  sauce

... FOR QUICK DINING

Clear vegetable soup
Spicy mushroom slices

Stuffed artichoke
Spicy tomato salad

Onion soup
Tasty croissants

Minestrone
Stuffed tomatoes from warmer
  regions

Artichoke soup
Steamed vegetables

Minestrone (without cheese)
Raw vegetable bread roll

Avocado soup
Bread with leek ragoût

... FOR FRUIT LOVERS

Fruity cheese sticks
Stuffed pineapple (without cream)

Stuffed pear on a bed of
  strawberries
Winter pineapple

Cinnamon apples
Stuffed pineapple (without cream)

Citrus salad
Layers of fruit salad

Stuffed apricots
Summer fruit with forest-fruit
  sauce

Avocado mousse
Fruit salad

Blanched pears with marjoram
Pineapple salad with coconut

BIBLIOGRAPHY

J. Dries: *The Acid-Base Balance*, Arinus, 1991

J. Dries: *Dietetics*, Arinus, 1988

J. Dries: *Foodtherapy*, Arinus, 1990

J. Dries: *Natural Food for Daily Use*, Arinus, 1978

Prof.-Dr F. van Faassen: *Anatomie, Histologie en Fysiologie van de Mens*, Samson Stafleu, Alphen aan de Rijn/Brussels, 1986

Prof.-Dr M. Cokelaere: *Functionele Anatomie van de Mens*, Parts 1 and 2, Aurelia, St.Martens-Latem, 1986

W. Kahle, H. Leonhardt and W. Platzer: *Sesam Atlas van de Anatomie*, Part 2, Bosch & Keuning, Baarn, 1986

Stefan Sibernagl and A. Despopulos: *Sesam Atlas van de Fysiologie*, Bosch & Keuning, Baarn, 1987

J. A. Bernards and L. N. Bouman: *Fysiologie van de Mens*, Bohn, Scheltema & Holkema, Utrecht/Antwerp, 1983

J. F. de Wijn and W. T. J. M. Hekkens: *Fysiologie van de Voeding*, Bohn, Scheltema & Holkema, Utrecht/Antwerp, 1989

Dr W. Stortenbeek: *Het Zuur-Base Evenwicht bij de Mens*, Bohn, Scheltema & Holkema, Utrecht/Antwerp, 1979

Prof.-Dr M. Joniau: *Algemene en Menselijke Biochemie*, Acco, Louvain, 1976

Dr F. Smet and Dr P. Lambers: *Biochemie*, Bohn, Scheltema & Holkema, Utrecht/Antwerp, 1986

C. H. Gray and P. J. Howorth: *Biochemie Pathologie*, De Tijdstroom, Lochem-Poperingen, 1981

P. Karlson, W. Gerok and W. Gross: *Pathobiochemie*, George Thierne Verlag, Stuttgart, 1982

Dr W. Batles: *Lebensmittelchemie*, Springer Verlag, Berlin, 1983

Dr H. Geesing: *Die Beste Waffe des Körpers – Enzyme*, Herbig, Munich, 1990

G. Leibold: *Enzymen*, De Driehoek, Amsterdam, 1986

Dr G. J. H. den Ottolander: *Interne Geneeskunde*, Bohn, Scheltema & Holkema, Utrecht/Antwerp, 1989

Dr L. Wendt: Die *Eiweisspeicherkrankheiten*, Haug Verlag, Heidelberg, 1979

Dr E. Rauch: *Diagnostik Nach Dr Mayr*, Haug Verlag, Heidelberg, 1979

Dr Z. Cope: *Vroege Diagnostiek van Acute Buikaandoeningen*, Bohn, Scheltema & Holkema, Utrecht/Antwerp, 1982

Prof.-Dr H. Mehnert: *Prof.-Dr H. Förster: Stoffwechselkrankheiten*, George Thierne Verlag, Stuttgart, 1975

W. Nultsch: *Algemene Botanie*, Parts 1 and 2, Het Spectrum, Utrech/Antwerp, 1976

A. Quispel and D. Stegwee: *Plantenfysiologie*, Bohn, Scheltema & Holkema, Utrecht/Antwerp, 1983

Dr Ludwig Walb: *Die Haysche Trennkost*, Haug Verlag, Heidelberg, 1971

Dr L. Walb and Dr T. Heintze: *Het Hay-diet*, De Driehoek, Amsterdam, 1991
Dr Herbert M. Shelton: Dutch translation *Gezond Eten Door Juiste Voedselcombinaties*,
    Nieuw Leven, Genk, 1978
Bässler, Fekl. Land: *Grundbegriffe der Ernährungslehre*, Springer Verlag, Berlin 1979
Dr J. F. de Wijn and Dr W. A. van Staveren: *De Voeding van Elke Dag*, Bohn
    Scheltema & Holkema, Utrecht/Antwerp, 1984
Prof.-Dr M. Cokelaere: *Praktische Voedingsleer*, Aurelia, St.Martens-Latem, 1983
Prof.-Dr M. Cokelaere: *Algemene Voedingsleer*, Aurelia, St.Martens-Latem, 1987
Dr Herbert M. Shelton: German translation *Richtige Ernährung*, Waldthausen Verlag,
    Rittenhude, 1989
G. Liebster: *Warenkunde Obst und Gemüse*, Parts 1 and 2, Morion, Dusseldorf, 1991
Prof.-Dr Paul Mori: *Das Naturgesetz der Ernährung*, H. Schwab Verlag, Geinhausen,
    1962
T. L. Cleave: *Krank Durch Zucker und Mehl*, Bioverlag Gesundleben, Hopferau, 1983
H. W. Goll: *Milchsäure*, Reformhaus Fachakademie, Oberursel, 1988
Prof.-Dr R. Wenger: *Diätetik*, Springer Verlag, Wenen, 1964
Jan Dries: *Natuurvoeding Voor Dagelijks Gebruik*, Nieuw Leven, Genk, 1986
L. Schlegel: *Rohkost und Rohsäfte*, Hippokrates Verlag, Stuttgart, 1956
Prof.-Dr P. de Moor and Dr A. Hendrickx: *Moderne Dieetleer*, Stafleu's
    Wetenschappelijke Uitgeverij, Leiden, 1968

SOURCES OF ANALYTICAL DATA

Die Grosse GU Nährwert Tabelle (nutrition charts), Institute for
Nutritional Research at the Universities of Vienna and Giessen, 1992–3

Dutch foodstuffs data: Voorlichtingsbureau voor de Voeding (Nutritional
Information Bureau), The Hague, 1990

Belgian foodstuffs data: Nubel VZW, Brussels, 1992

R. S. K. Werte, Flüssiges Obst Verlag, 1987

Confructa Studien, Rohwarenkunde für die Fruchtsaftenindustrie, Flüssiges
Obst Verlag, 1985

Acid contents and pH values of foods: Jan Dries, 1992

SUBJECT INDEX

RECIPE INDEX

APPETIZERS

SOUPS

SALADS

PASTA AND RICE DISHES

BREAD ROLLS AND TOASTS

CHEESE DISHES

DRESSINGS AND SAUCES

NON-ALCOLHOLIC BEVERAGES